The Mystery of
Alzheimer's

Elizabeth Forsythe was born in London in 1927, studied medicine at King's College, London and King's College Hospital Medical School and qualified in 1950. Her experience in medicine has included general practice, psychiatry, public health and family planning, her professional work fitting in around her marriage and three children. She has travelled widely and lived and worked in Switzerland, the Highlands of Scotland and in East Anglia.

She started in journalism more than thirty years ago and has contributed to many publications including the *Scotsman* and, more recently, *Choice* magazine. She has also written a number of books, one of which was on Alzheimer's disease, from which her husband died in 1986: *Alzheimer's Disease; the Long Bereavement* (Faber & Faber, 1990) won the top award of the Medical Journalists' Association in 1991. She edited the last two editions of *Faber's Pocket Medical Dictionary* and for seven years the *British Journal of Family Planning*. Elizabeth Forsythe now lives and writes in rural East Anglia, and has completed her first novel.

Dr Elizabeth Forsythe

The Mystery of Alzheimer's

A Guide for Carers

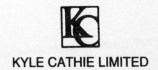

KYLE CATHIE LIMITED

First published 1996 by
Kyle Cathie Limited
20 Vauxhall Bridge Road
London SW1V 2SA

ISBN 1 85626 220 0

A CIP catalogue record for this title
is available from the British Library

Typeset by SX Composing DTP
Printed and bound by Cox & Wyman, Reading Berks.

FOR MY CHILDREN AND GRANDCHILDREN

Acknowledgements

I thank the narrators on both sides of the Atlantic, FG, KW, JB, MC, FC and WS, who gave so generously of their time, thought and feelings to give the accounts of those near them who had, or had had, Alzheimer's disease. I thank my friends Canon Denis Payne, Dr Ruth Skrine, Sheila Upjohn and Julia Cleave who, during these years of quest have, in varied and distinct ways, been my guides, mentors, inspirers and encouragers, and to Mark Warner, Alan Pegg and Steve Harnden who in practical ways have enabled me to write this book. I thank my friends at Apple Farm, Michigan, for allowing me to quote from Helen Luke's essays *Old Age*, published by Parabola Books, and Peter Brook, for his permission to quote from his essays in *There Are No Secrets*, published by Methuen. And I thank Kyle Cathie and her team for their help and the freedom they have allowed me in the writing of this book.

CHAPTER 1

The Start of a Quest

My husband John died from Alzheimer's disease in 1986. In the decade since his death I have spent much of my time and resources in an attempt to understand this strange and devastating disease which gradually destroyed him and caused havoc in the relationships around him. My medical training influenced me to start this search along orthodox lines, asking such questions as what is Alzheimer's disease and who is or was Alzheimer? What has happened in the brains of those who develop it? How does it start? What are the causes? What about the possibility of treatment? What is the best sort of management? Will it ever be cured? Then my questioning has gone further, to wanting to know more about the sort of people who do and do not develop the disease. And, as I move into my old age, how can I live so that I do not disintegrate in this way? During this quest I have had a recurring sense of the inadequacy of the present state of affairs.

This is not a practical handbook about how to care for somebody who is already ill with this sickness, nor is it a scientific investigation. Orthodox medical research tends to concentrate on what has happened, and how one can recognise Alzheimer's disease by various tests. My own inner promptings have led me further back, to questions about why this has happened, and what one can possibly do so that it will not happen. Having edited an orthodox medical journal for seven years, I am acquainted with the rigours of medical research, of double-blind controlled trials, and of having sufficient numbers in any trial to make the conclusions valid. Here I am breaking every scientific rule, but I know that I am doing so. I am taking a leap into a different understanding of the disease, by looking in detail at the narratives of six people, three in the UK and three in America. Through these narratives I attempt to understand the disease, not in terms of physical changes, but through the personality and family background of the patient.

The story of John

During the last ten years of John's life, I knew that he was changing but did not understand what was happening to him. In spite of my own medical training, and some years' experience in psychiatry, I did not understand that he was developing Alzheimer's disease. After his retirement he went each year for a private medical check and was apparently reported as healthy. It was only many years later that I discovered that, on each occasion, his mental state was queried but his doctor did not see the point of raising the matter with him.

My initial reaction to his sickness was that it was a disease, and that there must be an identifiable cause. I can remember driving to see him during the summer of 1985, at a time when Alzheimer's disease certainly seemed a possibility. I drove along a road with brilliant rapeseed oil plants on either side, listening to a programme about Alzheimer's disease on my car radio. It was about aluminium, and the reasons why it was a likely cause of this sort of dementia. I jumped at this explanation of all the problems confronting me at that moment. I thought of the large amounts of indigestion mixture, headache remedies and hangover medicines that John had taken over many years, all containing aluminium. We did not have aluminium saucepans, but I realised that, if we had, I should be at equal risk of developing dementia. But I never took any of those medicines, and at that moment this seemed confirmation of the idea that aluminium had caused John's Alzheimer's disease. I had a great sense of relief that I now understood the disease. The world brightened a little. I did know that the course of John's illness was not likely to be changed by my current knowledge, or the removal of all the aluminium-containing medicines from his daily intake, but I had a fleeting sense of certainty. That is what I needed to help me cope while faced with an unknown set of events, and my fear and apprehension. No human being likes to be confronted with something he cannot understand and feels unable to control. I was no exception, in spite of a medical training and experience in psychiatry.

During the following year, until his death in October 1986, there was little comfort to be found in that fleeting moment of certainty. I did not do the practical day-to-day caring because of the breakdown of the family early in 1981, but I had to bear the brunt of John's disintegration and accept the responsibilities which it involved. During that year of confusion I had support from a remarkable solicitor, a dependable contact at the Court of Protection and, during John's last months, an able and wise young general practitioner. I mention these firm, supportive people here because, over the years that I have puzzled over the meaning of this strange and frightening disease, I have realised that however much we relatives and carers want simple scientific

answers, in the end it is human resources that provide enduring remedies.

John could never have written his own story at any time
in his life. During my quest in the years since his death I have
realised that nobody who dies from Alzheimer's disease
could write the story of his own life without much outside
help. Harold Wilson, the former British Prime Minister,
died from the disease in 1995. Although he was a scholar and
author of historical and political books he did not write an
autobiography. It was announced in 1995 that Ronald
Reagan, the former President of the United States, is also ill
with Alzheimer's disease; he has not written an autobiography. I watch with interest other retired politicians and
wonder if any autobiography they write has a ghost writer. I
realised that I must attempt to understand, by a great effort
of imagination, what it is in the person who develops
Alzheimer's disease that makes it impossible for him to tell
his own story. Is it something lacking inside him? Is it
because of an early training? I also ask myself if the person
who develops Alzheimer's disease could ever have written
his own story, and is there any possibility that I could write
it from the patient's point of view. Ultimately I shall have to
see my own way.

For many of us, increasing age and more leisure give us
the time and opportunity to look at our lives, see them with
experienced eyes, and begin to have a clearer idea about
who and what we are, what meaning our lives have, what
our lives have meant to us and those closest to us, what their
lives have meant to us and, most important of all, to distinguish who we are from what we have done and achieved.
John could never have thought or talked about such things.
There were large parts of his life which were always secret.

I believe they remained hidden even from himself. In an extraordinary way, his death from Alzheimer's disease was a logical end to his fragmented and hidden life. There seemed no possibility that he and his life could have been made whole.

John was born in Surrey in 1910 and was an only child. His father, Robin, was born in India because his father, Jock, was in the army, stationed there. Robin's mother died when a younger brother was born, two years after his own birth. The two small boys remained in India and were brought up by servants until they came to back to the United Kingdom when Robin was about eight years old. They were then educated privately in Ireland. When Jock retired from the army, Robin went to live with him at the family home in Scotland and went to work in the office of a cousin who was a Writer to the Signet. However, Robin gave up any idea of entering the legal profession and spent three years in the Scottish Customs and Excise. He started writing poetry and had some published in the Glasgow Weekly Herald. He moved to London and tried his hand at freelance journalism and short-story writing. His first efforts were discouraging but he then had short stories published and won two awards. He started writing mystery thrillers which were published by the Bodley Head; some were translated into French. He also did watercolour paintings and conté portraits which were exhibited in London. Robin married in 1906, John was born in 1910 and in about 1920 Robin and his wife separated, although they seem to have been together again during the last years of his life. He died in 1937 at the age of fifty-seven.

Robin Forsythe seems to have been an outstandingly intelligent and creative man but probably a loner. John never spoke about his father and it is only from scraps of paper I have found written by Robin for publishers that I know anything about him. It was as though John preferred to deny rather than acknowledge and delight in his own artistic inheritance. He confirmed this denial by getting rid of most of his father's paintings and drawings in the autumn of 1980. Possibly his father's artistic temperament contributed to the breakdown of his parents' marriage. I think that John was temperamentally, as well as physically, like his father, and a shy and sensitive child who suffered during his parents' separation. From the age of ten he was brought up in Glasgow by his mother and three of her childless sisters.

His ambition had been to study engineering and at seventeen he started a course in London. But under pressure from family and friends, and with the incentive of more money and better prospects, he went into a business of fibre-brokers in London. He was able, in this job, to use his considerable talents for learning, speaking and working in a variety of foreign languages. I think that he was always a solitary person, although at times he seemed superficially to want to be with a lot of people. During the 1939–45 war his talent for languages was put to good use in the secret intelligence service in a number of postings attached to various embassies. This helped him develop an easy manner in getting on with a great variety of people, as well as a talent for travelling and entertaining. These skills were of use to him later in his business life. His inner solitariness was protected by this outer veneer of sociability and gregariousness. He had few close friends but many acquaintances. By the end of his life his solitariness was paramount. During his dementia he was completely isolated and it was impossible for anybody to reach him.

When we married he was forty-five and I was seventeen

years younger. My enjoyment of closeness and warmth in relationships probably attracted him to me in the first place because these emotions had been absent in his life. He was very tall and dark and his mother was exceptionally small and fair. I was then also tall and dark haired, and now that I look at photographs of his father, I resembled him very much more than his mother. I never knew John's father but in character, and in artistic talents, I think that I resembled him. At that time I had not even seen a photograph of his father (he had died nearly twenty years previously) and neither John nor his mother spoke about Robin. It is only recently that I have been aware how strange it is that John was attracted to somebody who must, at a deep level, have brought back repressed memories of his father. I believe that years later, when his dementia had started, his rejection of me was an echo of his rejection of, and possibly by, his father.

John was always a little remote, but I found that attractive and was fascinated by his remarkable talent with languages and his ability to adapt to different countries and to the varying roles in his life. He was a successful businessman and much esteemed by his colleagues, yet there was always the sense that he was acting a role and did not see himself as a businessman. He had expensive and immaculately tailored business suits but would then wear a shabby tweed coat over the top and a rather battered felt hat or, at weekends, a beret. This contradiction between the desire to be totally conventional and a secret desire to be very unconventional, or even eccentric, ran through all his life. He wanted the presence of a wife, and the appearance of an established and 'happy' home life, without the need to be committed to it or to make any effort to work to support the image. He was pleased to have children but avoided any responsibility in being a father. There was always this contradictory strand of wanting to make the right appearance, give a proper impression and play a correct role in all the different spheres of his life, but at the same time he avoided the commitment that could bring reality or meaning to any of his relationships.

My emotional reactions attracted him initially, but later terrified him, and our marriage became, for the most part, a distant relationship of varying roles. He was away travelling for business during a third of the year and worked long days when he was at home. He had the use of a flat in London and when he was particularly hard-pressed in the office or involved in business entertaining he stayed there. I seldom joined him for entertaining in London because we had three children but sometimes guests came home and I enjoyed entertaining them. It was always a strain because everything had to be done perfectly and achieved without any hitches and that could be difficult with small children. However, I liked the challenge, and feared his annoyance if anything went wrong.

I shall never know what our relationship meant to him. Our happiest times together were while travelling, either for pleasure or work. When the children were older I did travel with him on a number of occasions. Perhaps when we were travelling we were both equally removed from the realities of looking after a home and bringing up children and could therefore share a world, for a limited time, on equal terms. I could give him all my time and attention. I always hoped that one day these intervals of peace which I enjoyed, and he seemed to enjoy as much, would be extended into what I always saw as our 'real' life at home with our family, but those hopes were not fulfilled.

John's paternal grandmother, who had died in childbirth in India, had come from Caithness. This connection, and an expatriate Scot's longing to return to his roots and 'homeland', encouraged him to buy land in Caithness in 1969. I do not know if, when he bought it, he had any particular intention of moving there, but he had vague ideas that one day he would have the time and money to do different things. He thought about working with wood. Turning wood interested him more than carving, but he had a longing to do something with his hands and create something other than making money.

Looking back now, nearly ten years after John's death and more than twenty years since his vague desires to find his true home took place in reality, I understand more about the meaning of his search. For the majority of human beings, particularly in their later years, and particularly for those who have identified strongly with their achievements in the outer world, there is this strong desire to find a real homeland. During my quest for the meaning of Alzheimer's disease, while I have listened intently to the narratives of those who have been close to a victim, I have heard about this search repeatedly.

It seemed so important that John should find his roots in what he saw as his native land that I encouraged him in his hunt to find land in Caithness and, eventually, to build there a permanent home for the family. I felt sure that this was what he wanted and what was good for him must inevitably be good for me and the children. I am an intuitive person, but the intuitive person needs to know, and be reminded at frequent intervals, that her intuitions will be wrong as often as they will be right! At that time I had no understanding at all of the deeper meaning of a search for a real home.

In 1969 we bought land and ruins in the far north-east of Scotland and in due course, and with considerable difficulty, built a beautiful house overlooking a harbour and the Moray Firth. I moved up there with our three children, then fourteen, twelve and eleven, in 1973. At the time it seemed the best compromise. It was the best time to interrupt the children's education and John said that he intended to retire and come and live there in 1974. Sadly, many things happened to change those plans, including changes in his firm, and John did not retire until five years later. During those five years he lived his own life in the south of England, centred on his work in London. I think in those years he began to live out a fantasy. The split between his real world and all the might-have-beens or could-have-beens increased.

It is difficult to look back on the life of somebody who develops Alzheimer's disease and be able to say with any certainty 'Yes, it started at such and such a time', or even at about a certain time. This was so in John's life. Now, with the benefit of hindsight, it is possible to see markers along the way and changes and developments in his life that point towards his final disintegration. Also, with the benefit of hindsight, it is easy to say that John was not at all the same person outwardly when he retired in 1978 as he was when we made the decision to move to the far north of Scotland in 1969. I am sure that, when he did retire, his normal solitariness had tipped into an abnormal sort of isolation which progressed into dementia and disintegration. During the years that we lived mostly apart, separated by seven hundred miles, I had a hunch that there was another woman in his life but he never spoke about it and it seemed better to deny my hunch because of the many practical difficulties.

Early in 1978, while John was still working in London and living in our former home near Cambridge, he suddenly developed a severe pain in his back. He stayed in bed for a number of days and was seen by his general practitioner who could not make a diagnosis and did not give him anything to relieve the pain. After about a week, John decided to make the long journey north and arrived on the night sleeper in Inverness exhausted, in a lot of pain and depressed. He was glad to see me at the railway station. I had arranged for him to be admitted to an orthopaedic ward in Inverness for diagnosis and treatment. After a week he was discharged, in more or less the same state physically, and he came home to Caithness for a period of rest. Certainly he was in pain and much distressed about that, but he was also, quite uncharacteristically, depressed and tearful. He did not want me out of his sight. He kept saying that he had spent all his life worrying about his possessions and making money and he had ignored people. He was very sad that he had had so little time for his family during his working life, particularly during the previous five years. It was true that he had seldom come north and had seen little of me and his adolescent children. During these weeks he slept badly and was constantly preoccupied with his feelings of sadness. He said that all he wanted now, and for the rest of his life, was the time to spend with me and his family and to have the opportunities to make up for the estrangement in the past many years. It was a sad and distressing time but at the same time I could see this moment as holding great hope for the future.

I look back and see this as a time when John was on the point of picking up a new responsibility for his life, when he had an opportunity to make real relationships with those around him. At last he was going to retire. There would be a chance for him to do some of the things that he had said he wanted to do, and there would be time to do all the things together that we had talked about. For me there was an almost unbelievable feeling of relief that all the problems and isolation and rejection of past years might be dissipated. The move north had not been in vain and there was a real sense of hope for a different life in the future.

John's back became less painful and he decided to return to work in London full-time for six weeks before the end of July, which was the official date of his retirement. When he returned to the south he saw his own doctor again and was advised to see a physiotherapist privately to get treatment for his pain. At the time this advice seemed surprising because the pain had almost gone. I now think the pain could have been understood on various levels. For John there must have been intense pain at abandoning a lifetime of achievement and beginning to make relationships with those around him. I am sure that, for the time he had been in Scotland, that was his intention. It must have seemed a relief to accept physical treatment to take the whole problem away.

I do not know if those months prior to his return to London, a time that seemed to hold the key to great changes in him and in our future life together, were the time of onset of Alzheimer's disease. Certainly, something profound and disturbing was happening in John's mind. For many weeks we were extraordinarily close in sharing his sadness and our hopes. It seemed to be a turning point in his life and in our relationship. For years after his dementia and death, I wondered if any help could have made those potential changes into a continuing reality. I shall write more about these thoughts in the last two chapters of the book.

After he left for London, I did not see John again until his official retirement party. When we did meet, he was once again a distant stranger, and there was no more talk of our future plans nor of spending more time together. He stayed for a few more days in the south and then returned to Caithness. In 1972 he had bought an old Orkney sailing boat and had looked forward to renovating and then sailing it. Now he got involved in litigation with the boatyard that was doing some of the major repairs and it was many months before that was concluded and the boat was back in the harbour below our house and he could work on it. He would spend many hours getting ready to do a job on the boat and would take several car loads of tools and paints down to the harbour. Often, by the time that he was organised and had found appropriate clothes, it was time to start clearing up again. He seemed to be constantly active and occupied but, at the end of a day, had achieved nothing. I thought that this was another manifestation of the distress that he had shown earlier in the year and that it would pass as he settled down in his retirement. There was no time to go for a walk together or have lunch out because he was driven by his constant busy-ness.

In retrospect, an indication of his worsening condition was his attitude to money. John had a substantial 'golden handshake' from his firm when he retired. During his weeks at home, early in 1978, he had told me about the money and said that he intended to put part of it into two trusts, one to pay for the university education of our children and the other for an annuity for me, because his work pension made no provision for a widow and, with our age difference, it was likely that I should outlive him. When he returned from London he spoke no more about these financial provisions. John had always been mean and secretive about money until the earlier months that year, when he had sounded more generous. When the two older children started at university, in the autumn of 1978, John said that he did not have enough money to help them. He did not mention again his capital sum or the plans he had talked of earlier.

I had never known what his financial position was or how much money he earned. After the move to Caithness, I had always been short of money and did some journalism and part-time medicine to help pay the household bills. His sudden announcement that he was not able to make any contribution to our children's upkeep at university came as an amazing blow. I could think of no way in which I could support them. They applied for grants but were turned down.

It felt as though a door that had begun to open had slammed shut, or that the stranger with some sense of familiarity had gone and a stranger with a chilling feel of remoteness had arrived in his place. I found myself alone, very far from relatives and friends of long standing, with somebody who apparently wished to be entirely isolated, both physically and emotionally. The shock was greater because of the changes that I had glimpsed during the early months of that year. I became full of fear for him, for the children, for myself and for the future. At the time, I saw him as an unreasonable tyrant and I was afraid of him.

John believed that I was responsible for the problems he had in his retirement and he blamed it on the fact that I was English. Before his retirement, however, my Englishness had been graciously accepted by the local community. There was nobody at all at that time with whom I could discuss the whole painful situation. Had he really changed or was I different? Was there any way of escape from this nightmare? I could not find one and, at the end of 1980, I had a severe breakdown and was admitted to a mental hospital.

John said that he wanted a divorce and did not want me to come home again. By this time it was clear to him, and probably to me, that I was the one with a problem. After three months in hospital I returned to the south on my own, without job, money, home, family, husband, possessions or any understanding of what had happened. It was a time of great confusion for me. It did not occur to me that John might be mentally disturbed because I had accepted that I was the one with a mental illness. It was to be a number of years before I could begin to understand that there was any need or reason to help John. Fortunately I had good friends in the south and I survived.

From then on John made no contact with me. The following year he sold the house in Scotland and moved to a London suburb to be near his cousin. He did not send me any money from the sale of the house, which he had previously agreed to do. However, I managed to get part-time work. I rented an agricultural cottage and the children continued at university without any financial support from John. John did not let me know his new address or telephone number. I had no understanding of what had happened and eventually I tried not to think about him. I had to use my energy to struggle with my own depressive illness and demanding work.

When I wrote an account of this time in my first book on Alzheimer's disease, three years after his death, I was not able to disentangle my life and story from his. The book was muddled and the publishers asked me to rewrite it. This rewriting helped me in that aim. This was an example, not only of the difficulty of disentangling the story of a person from the history of the disease, but also of the destructive and engulfing effects of a partner's disintegration on the person who is emotionally closest. I could not distance myself from John sufficiently to see him clearly and objectively. He had always offloaded his problems onto somebody else; I had always not only felt responsible for my own shortcomings but also been prepared to shoulder his. Neither of us had any insight into the effects that the changes in him were having on me and our relationship. I was almost unaware of the subtle differences in John that were markers of his deterioration. It is difficult to distinguish between what is normal and difficult in a relationship, and when a boundary has been crossed and outside help is needed. It is easier to get outside help when the label of a disease can be put on the person.

Two years later our son graduated from Edinburgh University. He wanted both his parents to be present at his graduation ceremony. Peter had seen John at various times and thought that he was a bit difficult and demanding. He asked me to organise the day because he doubted his father's ability to do it. I was shocked when I met John because he seemed much older and was totally preoccupied with his poor eyesight, convinced that he was going blind. (He had always had healthy eyes.) John and I spent the afternoon together and walked back to the hotel where I was staying. For me, these hours together, which I knew were of limited duration, had a dreamlike quality. I was able to enter into John's world and appreciate it as he saw it.

It was a very frightening world. John believed that he was being pestered by people demanding money from him and sending him bills for things which he had never had. I do not know if, at the time, I thought that was the truth. I could understand that that was the way in which he saw his world and, strange as it seemed to me, it was entirely real for him.

In Caithness I had felt threatened by his strange view of reality but now I was no longer dependent on him, the physical and emotional distance made my understanding and acceptance of him greater. His obsession with money and belief that he was being hounded by people to pay debts for which he was not responsible were a further result of the drastic changes which took place in him in 1978.

John had no interest in what I or other family members were doing. I saw him that afternoon as a very sad and lonely person. I assured him that at no time would I ever ask for any financial help, but that assurance did not appear to give him any relief. I suggested that he might like to meet me sometimes in London and talk. He said that he would like that, but he would still not give me his address or telephone number. He said he would contact me.

He did not, and I did not see him again for another two years. By that time he no longer knew who I was. The meeting in Edinburgh could have been an opportunity for some sort of intervention. Sadly, I did not use it in this way to help him because I did not recognise the enormity of his disturbance. I also doubt if any intervention would have been acceptable to him.

A year later Peter was trying to equip a flat and asked John if he had any surplus household things for his bedroom and kitchen. John suggested Peter brought a van and met him at the garage outside his flat. However, when Peter arrived, John said he could give him very little because all his possessions had been stolen. Obviously this was extremely unlikely and was part of what, medically, could be called his delusions of poverty and persecution. Peter told me of this incident but I failed to understand the true nature of what was happening and thought John was just being ungenerous and possibly devious. Again there was confusion between the usual secretiveness and miserliness of John's personality and the changes which were now overt delusions. It was a further sign of his retreat into a private fantasy world and a strange and frightening life of total solitariness. This progression was so slow and subtle that I could not identify a time at which it was no longer 'normal' for John but some kind of recognisable disease.

The crisis in John's dementia, when intervention was unavoidable, came in the summer of 1985. He drove his car from a minor road into a major road without stopping, and hit a woman's car. He seemed unaware of the accident and drove on. The police went to his flat to interview him but probably realised that he was not able to give evidence and finally dropped any charges against him. The police notified his insurance company and confiscated his driving licence. I have noticed that the police often take an action that initiates the way to a diagnosis of Alzheimer's disease. The law has clear boundaries, and it is easier for a policeman to identify the crossing of such a boundary than for a doctor to recognise subtle changes in personality. John had been making his own rules for so many years that this brush with an outer, legal reality had a profound impact.

His cousin got in touch with me and wanted me to go and see him. I had not previously been to John's flat, but when I finally made the journey it was immediately identifiable by all the locks, spy-holes on the door and chalk-written signs and messages about where to put things. I rang the bell and could hear John walking around inside. It was ten minutes before he came to the door. I could see him looking through first one and then the other spy-hole. He finally opened the door a crack while it was still chained. He did not appear to recognise me and was very suspicious. I kept talking, with an ease I did not feel, and eventually he let me in. It was the middle of a rather hot afternoon but all the curtains were drawn, some of the windows were shuttered and the heating was on. John was partly dressed. He took me all the way through the flat to the furthest room, which was his bedroom. It was blacked out with curtains and black-out curtains, the electric lights were on and it was overpoweringly hot. The room was in a chaotic state, the bed was unmade and the sheets were dark with filth. The room smelt strongly of unwashed humanity. He told me to sit down and indicated one of the two large leather-covered director chairs in the room. Then he told me not to sit down but to put a towel on the seat first. He sat down on his bed and talked in jumbled sentences.

He watched me with a puzzled expression but without recognition. He got up, went to a shelf and picked up a photograph of me. He brought it over and thrust it at me, as a small child would, and told me that was Elizabeth. I tried to explain it was a photograph of Elizabeth and that was me, his wife. He did not seem able to put these two ideas together. He said that he had to go through to the other section to cut the hair on his face. He went to the bathroom but kept returning to comment on the difficulties of shaving. I had the feeling that he also needed to check up that I was still there. I was amazed to see about fifteen clocks in his bedroom but not one told the right time. There were two desks and piles of dirty papers, books and clothes lying in heaps on the bed and floor. From one of the walls was a branching column of electrical adapters about twelve inches long, with numerous side-branches, plugs and various radios, record players, calculators and other devices attached. They were all so dirty that it did not look as though they had been used recently.

I was appalled by the sights and smells and could only bear to stay there by trying to think with the medical part of me. It was almost impossible to understand that this sad and mad old man was really John, my husband, and the person of whom I had been so afraid. It was then that I realised that his mind was dementing.

John continued to potter in and out of his bedroom from the bathroom and described the difficulties of putting on his tie. He was wearing a suit with a waistcoat and that also presented difficulties. I offered to help, but he wanted to dress himself. Finally, when he was ready, we walked the short distance to his cousin's house. Two years previously he walked slowly; now he could barely shuffle. It was devastating.

During tea he kept up a loud childish prattle and repeatedly went off around the house to collect the possessions he had left there. At one point he had to be taken back to his flat to find a book he wanted to show me. He was behaving like a child but not at all like the solitary, quiet, shy child I had heard that he was. Now he was noisy, demanding of attention and constantly on the move. I wanted to do something to sort it all out but I knew that I was helpless, confused and inadequate. Here was my formidable husband acting like an anxious child.

John was in need of help. His cousin was a lonely person, after a series of bereavements, and liked to have John near her but she did not want to take responsibility for him. She probably realised that his condition was deteriorating but she wanted him to stay in his own flat. Nobody knew what his financial position was and so we could not employ help or begin to investigate the possibility of moving him into a home. I doubt if he could have been persuaded to accept either of these possibilities. I could see no way through this dilemma and went home feeling overwhelmed by the horror of the situation.

When I got home I telephoned John's doctor because I wondered if he had any ideas about what could be done. It was impossible to speak to him. I wrote and received no answer. After many attempts to speak to him on the telephone I did at least begin to know his receptionist. She was most helpful but could do nothing about John; the doctor remained elusive. John's cousin telephoned me frequently, often late at night, to say that it was impossible for her to cope and that I must do something. My mind ran in unproductive circles while I tried to think what I could do.

These months of confusion were certainly bad for John and they were also destructive for me and his family. John's cousin remained definite that she wanted him near. At the time I tried to keep the peace with her; I did not realise that her wishes had nothing to do with John and his welfare. I thought that it was impossible for me to do anything effective and of real help to John. I was wrong about my inadequacy. When I did, many months later, make positive decisions and initiate actions with John's good as my intention, I realised that there was a lot more I could have done earlier to relieve some of John's suffering. If his general practitioner had had some understanding of dementia and been able to meet me and discuss it with me it would have been helpful. Perhaps he was ignorant about dementia, or not interested or he felt it was inappropriate because I was not living with John.. A doctor must always put the best interest of his patient first but this would normally allow him to talk about the problems of a dementing patient with the nearest relative. It is possible that John's paranoia about his wife and family made it unlikely that his doctor would be willing to speak to his wife. As far as I know his cousin never attempted to make contact with his doctor.

In September 1985 I spent a few days on holiday with a wise friend whose mother had died from dementia. It was three days before I managed to speak about John because I felt so confused, distressed and guilty about him. She helped me enormously by telling me, among other things, about the power of attorney and the Court of Protection. This was my first contact with anybody who had commonsense and experience and knew some of the facts. My sense of hopelessness and confusion is, I now believe, part of the scenario of dementia. It is as though the confusion in the patient's mind spreads out at a hidden level to affect all those around, like the roots of one diseased tree infecting the neighbouring trees. The only sound way to deal with this insidious spreading infection is to get the facts. Good intentions and being kind to people do not help. Only facts, which can be looked at objectively and implemented when necessary, can begin to clear a path through the muddle.

During the next three months I went to see John as often as possible and tried repeatedly to get an appointment to see his doctor. I did find out about the Court of Protection but remained remarkably ignorant and confused about what I could or should do. Eventually I saw John's doctor. He confirmed that John's mental state had been queried at his medical checks and explained that, as there was nothing he, the GP, could do, he had not contacted him. He still saw no point in getting a psychogeriatrician to see John.

John started to wander at night and got lost on a number

of occasions. The police found him and took him back to his cousin. She telephoned me and told me to do something. I suggested that she should tell the police that she could not cope. But she would not do that and she refused to tell anybody, apart from me, the extent of the terrible state in which he was living. I went on procrastinating, and chaos continued.

Finally, I consulted a solicitor who was well informed and disciplined, knew the limits of what he could and could not do and, under his reserved manner, was a man of compassion. He was the first professional person I had met who was competent and could bring all the relevant matters together, jettison those that were irrelevant and begin to find some resolution. Meeting and speaking with him was for me a watershed, and a first step towards disentangling the conundrum. He started the proceedings for me to become the Receiver under the Court of Protection. John's doctor was asked to sign a form to say that John was not capable of managing his own affairs but he would not do this and the delay ran into months. I telephoned him and wrote to him but he would neither speak to me nor answer my letters. Eventually I persuaded John's doctor to arrange a domiciliary visit from a psychogeriatrician. I hoped that it might then be possible to get the papers signed for the Court of Protection. The visit took place and it was confirmed that John had some sort of dementia. The question of whether John should be sectioned and admitted temporarily to a mental hospital was discussed but no decision was taken. I was not there because I was ill.

The situation deteriorated and it became clear that John could no longer live on his own. The general practitioner signed the papers for the Court of Protection. The consultant saw John again, as did a social worker, and eventually he was sectioned and taken to a mental hospital. His cousin was much distressed and wanted him to come home again.

While John was in the mental hospital I managed to get to his flat and, with the help of a social worker, go through his papers and begin to get his financial affairs in some semblance of order. We realised that he could afford to go into a comfortable nursing home and I decided that, as John's cousin wanted him to be near her, we should look for a nursing home in that area. We found one which seemed to be good and comfortable. He could have a large ground-floor room with his own furniture, bathroom and door into a walled garden. It seemed a good solution and he was moved there.

Three weeks after John went there, the agreed fee rose sharply without any prior information. I was very surprised and felt acute unease which later showed itself to be justified. I contacted the nursing home and discovered it had changed hands. A medical friend told me about a recently opened mental nursing home in Norfolk which had an excellent reputation. I went to see it and was impressed with the management, the staff and the general atmosphere. The house and grounds were beautiful and, although there was no single room available, I arranged for John to be admitted three days later. Suddenly I knew what had to be done in his best interests. Having looked at the facts, I was sure about what I was doing and acted with urgency. It is sad that I had not had the same confidence to put John's interests of paramount importance long before this.

I arranged for a medical agency to move John the two hundred miles or so from one nursing home to the other.

The director thought that an ambulance might frighten him and sent his own car with two nurses, one of whom was a trained mental nurse; the other acted as driver. I went down with them. When I went into the nursing home I did not recognise John. He was almost rigid, he could barely shuffle, his saliva ran down his face and he was an unusual yellow colour. He looked like a living corpse. It was horrifying but I did not stop to discuss it with the staff. The most important thing now was to get him back to the quiet haven I had found for him in Norfolk. I wanted him near me, so I could see him regularly and know that he was being well looked after. The journey took about four hours but it seemed never-ending. He was so stiff that the nurses and I had to push him hard to bend him enough to sit in a car. I sat beside him on the back seat and kept looking to see if he was still breathing. It was difficult to see if he was or not. His face had no expression and the only sign of life was the slightest flicker of his eyelids from time to time.

In previous years we had spent a lot of time in Norfolk on holiday. As we started to drive through Thetford forest I was aware of some increase of life in John. He did not or could not move his head but his eyes seemed to be looking through the windows. I told him where we were and reminded him of all the previous times we had driven along that road. We arrived at the nursing home and he was welcomed and made comfortable. He seemed to enjoy his supper. The matron was horrified by the state he was in and thought that he had probably been given too many drugs. Their doctor later confirmed that he had drug-induced Parkinsonism.

John lived for another six months and I think, for much of that time, he was reasonably happy. At times I caught glimpses of a smile of recognition. I was, and remain, glad that, during those last months of his life, he was near enough for me to see him regularly. I think that it is important to spend time with somebody who is dementing, for your own sake even if they apparently do not recognise you. He did not know who I was, was doubly incontinent and had to be fed. Everything that I did for him during those months helped me to sort out my own confused feelings about him. In the simple acts of feeding him, or helping him dress, or sitting and holding his hand, or playing ball with a soft ball, I could recognise some of the tenderness I had felt in a previous time. I could start to accept all the paradoxical emotions of love and hate, anger, pity and despair.

John made a good recovery from the drug overdosage but, as he became more active, he was very spiteful. Sometimes he would do nothing but hit, pinch and bite. He did talk a little but it was almost impossible to understand anything he said. There was a memorable occasion when I went to see him wearing an old jacket which I had bought from an exclusive shop in a sale. His hand shot out and he said 'Nice piece of cloth'. It was his voice of many years before, and one of his skills had been the assessment of the quality of fibre yarns. It is strange that this skill, and the words that went with it, had survived with such clarity in a chaotic brain.

He needed a lot of care during the day and night and I was amazed at the skills and patience of the women care attendants in the nursing home. There was always a trained mental nurse on duty but most of the practical work was done by local girls and women from the surrounding villages, with no particular training but with the requisite gifts.

John's physical deterioration was rapid during the last

three months of his life and he shrivelled. He died in October 1986, two days before his birthday. Although he had not recognised me for more than a year, during his dying I know, beyond any shadow of doubt, that he did know me and understood something I needed to say to him before we were parted. His dying brought us back together again after many years of difficulty and much distress. His death was so peaceful and, in a surprising way, made some sense for me of all the tragedies of the preceding years.

Looking back now at John's life and death I see him as a pale floating person on his particular life's stage. He could be described as unrooted in his own life. So much of his past, his childhood, his ancestors are unknown. He never spoke of them and his artistic inheritance remained hidden.

CHAPTER 2

The guilt of the survivor and my quest for understanding

Following John's death, the confusion and distress continued and were more intensely painful than during his lifetime. At first I was numbed by my sense of guilt that he had died and that I had survived. When I wrote my first book about Alzheimer's disease, which was three years after his death, I was so ashamed of having survived that I gave the royalties away. I needed the money, but giving it away helped me to assuage some of my guilt. I am writing this book at the end of 1995; this year is the fiftieth anniversary of the ending of the 1939–1945 war. During the past months I have seen and heard many interviews with survivors of the holocaust and prisoner-of-war camps in which they have talked repeatedly about the unbearable feelings of guilt at having survived. This sense of guilt and need to appease has, on many occasions, stopped me making clear decisions. During my long and ongoing search for the meaning of Alzheimer's disease, I have realised that I am not the only close person to have been afflicted in this way. I now believe that these feelings are closely connected with the deep roots of Alzheimer's disease. Ultimately survival for the carer depends on her ability to distinguish herself from the patient at every level. An important first step in being able to make this distinction is to know the facts about the disease and to find out what can be done to support the patient and the carer during his lifetime and, after his death, the carer.

The patient and the carers

When the patient has reached the stage of disintegration when a medical diagnosis of Alzheimer's disease can be made, it is virtually unknown for there to be any reversal of the progressive decline and eventual death. That is a tragedy. However, it frequently occurs that the person most closely involved and most emotionally tied to the dementing person also becomes ill with depression, cancer, or sometimes dementia, and may predecease the patient. This is a double tragedy, but there may be ways in which this second tragedy can be prevented. The nature of Alzheimer's disease, and the strange way in which it subtly affects all those around the patient, make it important that some firm ground can be found for the carers. Contributing to my state of confusion over so long a time was my ignorance of the facts about the nature of the disease and the practical things that could be done to help my husband and myself. So here are some of the facts which I gradually unearthed, which helped me to cope during and after John's death.

Who was Alzheimer and what is 'his' disease?

Alois Alzheimer was a German professor of psychiatry. In 1906 he gave a report about one of his patients who had died in April of that year. He had first seen her in November 1901. She had a poor memory and had difficulty in finding words, she did not know where she was, had unpredictable behaviour and could not manage socially. That sounds like a description of somebody with Alzheimer's disease as we know it now, but she was only fifty-one when it was diagnosed. This was accepted as a new type of dementia, which started before old age and caused widespread changes in the brain which could be seen through a microscope after the patient's death. At the time it was hoped that identifying physical changes in the brain would be a way of understanding all mental disease, including manic depressive illness and schizophrenia.

Alzheimer also described multi-infarct dementia, which is caused by deficiencies in the blood supply to the brain. This type accounts for about 20 per cent of dementia. Alzheimer's disease is sometimes abbreviated to AD, multi-infarct dementia to MID and another type, described as senile dementia of the Alzheimer type, to SDAT.

Alzheimer's disease is the commonest type of dementia. Although it has the name 'Alzheimer's Disease' it is not a straightforward illness like chickenpox. There is no causative virus which can be identified and no physical mode of spread to be investigated and understood. Although knowledge increases about what happens in the brain during the condition, nobody yet knows the reasons for its occurrence. Scientists learn more about what has happened but nobody understands why it has happened.

What is meant by 'disease'?

The medical definition of disease implies a condition occurring in a body or mind which has been previously healthy.

Webster's Medical Dictionary defines health as 'the condition of an organism or one of its parts in which it performs its vital functions normally or properly: The state of being sound in body or mind.' Under the heading 'mental health' in the *Oxford Companion to the Mind*, the characteristics of the mentally healthy person are described as 'the capacity to co-operate with others and sustain a close, loving relationship, and the ability to make a sensitive, critical appraisal of oneself and the world about one and to cope with the problems of living'. This is a tall order and I question the number of people who can claim that they are in a state of mental health in the Western world at the present time!

John was never able to make a sensitive, critical appraisal of himself and the world about him. I do not believe that John was healthy for the early part of the last ten years or so of his life and was then afflicted by a disease. I think that, for many years, he had been in a state of dis-ease which eventually made him unable to sustain any relationship within himself or outside himself, or to cope with any of the challenges of daily living.

Sometimes it is valuable to look at the root meanings of words because those words often go further back in history than our current usage of them and can reveal deeper meanings. The word 'disease' is defined in the *Dictionary of Word Origins*: 'disease and malaise are parallel formations: both denote etymologically an impairment of ease or comfort. Disease comes from Old French *desaise*, a compound formed from the prefix *dis*, not, lacking and *aise*, ease, and in fact at first meant literally discomfort or uneasiness. It was only towards the end of the 14th century that this sense began to narrow down in English to sickness.' This concept of there being dis-ease, or a lack of harmony, within a person has, for me, an echo of the feelings I had when I was with John during his last year of life. Dis-ease could also be understood as the splitting apart of the person's mind and then his body, and also of his relationships with others, a more widespread and far flung dis-ease. Could dis-ease be different from a disease, a sickness, such as tuberculosis, that has a definable physical cause?

'Health', from the same dictionary has this definition. 'Etymologically, health is the state of being whole' and the verb 'heal' comes from the same source. The idea of becoming whole is different from the concept of being cured of a disease, having something undesirable taken away. Possibly the so-called 'disease' could even be part of a state of wholeness. It is tempting, in this scientific age, when it is normal to think in terms of problems to be identified and solved, to expect simple answers about the cause, cure and prevention of any disease. The word disease in its modern interpretation of 'sickness' does suggest that a cure will be possible, given enough scientific investigation. It also reinforces the idea that the disease is a distinct entity, separate from the person who has it. But if one thinks of dis-ease, it is possible to think of dementia as an integral part of the person who has it. There is not then a clear-cut distinction between the person and the dis-ease. The state of disintegration is very threatening, and with good reason, to those around. It involves a disintegration of the whole personality and the link between the old, normal, and the new, abnormal and disintegrated, state gets more blurred as the dis-ease progresses. This idea is important for carers to understand so that they may remain as objective as possible and maintain their own integrity.

My instinct told me this during and after John's death. I needed, on a number of occasions, to wear my 'medical hat' in order to have a sense of detachment. Then I was more able to make the best decisions for John and at the same time lay the foundations for my own survival.

In one sense, as soon as a condition is diagnosed as a recognisable disease it can be handed over to the doctor. The doctor or other therapist usually then prescribes a treatment and thus relieves the patient of the responsibility for his disease. This unspoken, unwritten deal is a legitimate piece of trading. The patient and the doctor collude in the belief that it is now the doctor's responsibility and not the patient's. A further step along this path leads to the unvoiced understanding that the doctor now has the power to deal with the sickness and remove it.

If Alzheimer's disease is a sickness like pneumonia, in due course the problem can be solved and a cure will be found. The diagnosis will be made by suitable investigations and scientific research will discover a drug to alter the damaged brain. There may be some elements of truth in this but I believe the whole truth is somewhere beyond this. I think of one person whose narrative is in this book, whose cousin concentrated on the physical minutiae. She was certain that if only the dementing person had a new set of false teeth, and could eat better, he would be better nourished and would then get better. Another relative was sure that, if the dementing patient had stronger glasses, he would be able to read and understand the printed word again. If he could read the newspaper, and understand what was in it, he would then speak sensibly as he always used to. She believed that all his mental confusion was caused by his poor glasses. There is a grain of truth in these ideas because, if somebody has a failure in hearing or vision and the incoming messages to the brain are incomplete or scrambled, there can be confusion in their reception by the brain. If somebody with failing hearing refuses to wear a hearing aid, or only wears it occasionally, he will never get the same benefit from it as somebody who knows his need and sets out to adapt to the aid. The old person who is deaf becomes isolated and sometimes believes that voices he is unable to hear are antagonistic to him. But, in the last analysis, we do not see with our eyes or hear with our ears. They are the channels which conduct the messages from the outer world to the correct bit in the brain where the messages are decoded. The messages do need to get in, as clearly as possible, but changing the strength of the glasses or the efficiency of a hearing aid will not help the dementing person to receive and understand incoming messages.

Alzheimer's disease, if seen as a series of physical failings, will be progressively handed over to health professionals, but a vision of the whole person and the meaning of the dis-ease will be lost. Late in John's life, when his legs were weak because his walking was affected by the progress of the dementia, he managed to say 'Need new legs. Go to leg shop. Get legs. Need new legs.' At one level he was right and did need new legs. He expressed the need and the solution in the way which had been most usual for him. If you needed something you bought it from the appropriate place. But on this occasion, buying a pair of legs would in no way help his condition. I believe that emphasis on the physical nature of the disease and attempts to patch up physical inadequacies, while at the same time denying the underlying mental state, hastens the ultimate disintegration of the whole person. I have recently heard of a person who is dementing and finds it difficult to walk. She is soon to have knee surgery. The real problem is her mental confusion; hospital admission and an anaesthetic will be harmful and not helpful to her mental state. I am not suggesting that age or physical need is a barrier to appropriate treatment, but I think it is important that there are clear decisions about what is the appropriate treatment for each individual.

Dementia and old age

Dementia is most commonly a disease of old age, but old age is certainly not the cause of dementia. Most people in older age forget the names of people and things. In medical language this is called nominal aphasia. It is as though the brain is occupied with other things, and the degree of this failing depends on fatigue and general health. Anxiety and fear about these failures in memory make the condition worse; conversely, explanation about its normality relieves the anxiety and tends to improve the condition.

Until the 1960s Alzheimer's disease was considered a rare disease, occurring in those under the age of sixty. When evidence of brain changes was more widely recognised, with the use of new electron microscopes, the whole conundrum of dementia became of greater scientific interest. In 1975 it was decided in America to discard the diagnosis of senile dementia and use the term Alzheimer's disease. From that time, the possibility of the state of dementia as dis-ease was less acceptable, and the idea of disease, with the possibility of a cure, was accepted.

Exact figures for the proportion of people in various age groups who become demented are difficult to ascertain, and the figures given in surveys in Europe and in the USA vary a great deal. The incidence increases with increasing age, and slightly more women than men are affected at all ages. It is more common in the USA than in Europe. Probably not more than 5 per cent of people between the ages of sixty-five and seventy are affected, but it rises to more than 20 per cent in those over eighty years of age. However, it is necessary to consider the criteria for diagnosis. It will never be easy to define accurately the number of dementing people in the population and it is likely to remain, to a certain extent, a hidden condition. The patient is very unlikely to be aware of his sickness, and the problem is most likely to be brought to a doctor's attention by relatives or friends, or when the nearest carer can no longer carry the burden. If there are many supportive people around the patient, or he lives in a close-knit community where his eccentricities can be tolerated, there may never be need to look for outside help.

There could be more than half a million people with Alzheimer's disease in the United Kingdom and the numbers are increasing, not because it is becoming a more common condition but because there is an increasing number of people surviving into old age. Our increased longevity is partly due to advances in medical care. For instance, bronchopneumonia, which has been described as 'the old man's friend', is now treatable and treated. More efficient influenza immunisations stop that disease spreading amongst vulnerable old people.

Causes of Alzheimer's disease

It is very difficult for us to live with questions, and it is normal to ask for answers even if they are incomplete. The word 'causes' assumes that this is a disease in the normal medical model, and for the moment I shall accept it as such. The cause remains elusive in spite of frequent reports of discoveries and breakthroughs. I doubt if any one cause will ever be found and, like other perplexing modern diseases, it will be understood as a multifactorial disease. The factors include the person's age, a genetic and/or a familial tendency, the patient's previous personality and possibly environmental factors.

It is important to understand the difference between the cause of a disease and correlations, or inter-relatedness, between the disease and a variety of factors, many of which will be characteristics of the people who get the disease. Advancing age correlates with the development of Alzheimer's disease, but getting older is not the cause of the disease. A few years ago there was a belief that aluminium was an important cause of Alzheimer's disease and, as I have explained, I jumped at this possibility at the time of John's diagnosis. Aluminium certainly never was thought to be the single cause of the disease, because it is a common element and we all drink and eat it, but we do not all get Alzheimer's. There is now good scientific evidence from Australia that aluminium can be exonerated. This type of oversimplification is unhelpful in the understanding of the disease and the only effect seems to be to increase distress. I think it is more likely that the use of aluminium saucepans is a common feature among the population that is now developing the disease. Aluminium saucepans were first in use after the First World War and those who were using them in the 1920s and 1930s are now coming into the age band for the onset of Alzheimer's. This is an example of a correlation and not a straightforward cause and effect relationship.

Genetic factors

The evidence that susceptibility to Alzheimer's disease may be genetically inherited strikes fear into the hearts and minds of those who are the blood relations of victims. It is a feeling of doom which is spoken in the old proverb, 'what's bred in the bone will come out in the flesh'. The evidence of a genetic inheritance needs critical appraisal. The clear-cut genetic inheritance described by the Austrian monk cum scientist, Gregor Mendel, in the nineteenth century gives a definite plan for the inheritance of certain traits, for example eye colour, from parents to their children. For many diseases, however, it is not so easy to identify the contribution that genetic inheritance plays.

There is stronger evidence of a genetic influence in a few families which have a pattern of presenile dementia; but these families are very rare. In other families there is a pattern of dementia through the generations but there is no clear evidence of genetic susceptibility. An enormous amount of research is now being done world-wide to find out which chromosomes are involved in the development of Alzheimer's disease. The aim is to find some way of preventing or changing the effects of the chromosomal abnormalities. There is an association between Down's syndrome and Alzheimer's disease; people with Down's syndrome frequently develop dementia if they live long enough. Research has concentrated on chromosome 21 which is involved in Down's syndrome. Chromosome 14 has been implicated in the common late-onset type of Alzheimer's disease and chromosome 19 is also being examined. All this remarkable research increases knowledge about the disease but it has little practical help to offer in the present management and treatment of the disease.

The idea that Alzheimer's disease is genetic can make an individual feel a helpless victim, but there may be other factors at work. It is possible that a repetition of family behaviour, through the generations, which can be disguised to the point of being difficult to recognise, could account for the reported figures that Alzheimer's disease is three times more likely to occur in first-degree relatives of people with both early- and late-onset Alzheimer's. If this is so, the individual has a greater degree of choice.

What happens in the brain?
Can the changes be controlled?

A great deal of research work is being done, with good financial backing from the pharmaceutical companies, to find ways of preventing the changes in the brain caused by Alzheimer's disease. If the onset could be delayed for five years it would be a considerable benefit for the patient, the carer and the resources of the health services.

During the course of the disease the brain shrinks. The surface of the normal brain has many nooks and crannies on it, but as the disease progresses the surface flattens out. Inside the normal brain there are spaces through which the cerebrospinal fluid circulates. These spaces expand during the disease. If the brain is examined after death, characteristic microscopic changes are found. Senile plaques are found outside the brain cell and on the surface of these cells is a protein called B-amyloid, which is normally embedded inside the brain cell. This protein is also laid down in the blood vessels in the body of somebody with Alzheimer's disease and probably accounts for the premature ageing. Neurofibrillary tangles are caused by abnormal deposits of protein in cells. The protein is necessary for the normal working of the brain but in Alzheimer's disease it gets overloaded with waste products and is unable to carry out its normal functions. It is thought that the presence of the neurofibrillary tangles predict the death of the cell.

The work of the brain is controlled by nerve cells, or neurons, and they communicate with each other by dendrites which pass electrical messages to the neighbouring cells. Between the cells there are gaps and messages have to get through these spaces using chemical substances called neurotransmitters. One of these is called acetylcholine and it is deficient in people with Alzheimer's disease. Acetylcholine is known to be involved in memory. Its shortage in Alzheimer's disease is caused by a deficiency in the enzyme responsible for making it. Twenty years after this discovery, a drug was developed in the USA to treat memory loss by increasing the levels of acetylcholine. Only a proportion of patients improved and some of those who did subsequently relapsed. It has not been licensed for use in the UK. Other lines of possible treatment by drugs are being followed up; each one is geared to one particular change found in the brain after death.

Other sorts of dementia

In multi-infarct dementia, the brain deteriorates because of a poor blood supply. The damage is patchy and the site of damage depends on where there is interference with the blood supply. The patient is usually known to have a high blood pressure and may have a history of strokes or mini-strokes shown by repeated short spells of giddiness or loss of consciousness. Sometimes these will be called TIAs, or transient ischaemic attacks. In multi-infarct dementia there are many small areas of deterioration in the brain and dementia may not be the first or only sign of damage. The progress of the disease is usually stepwise, which means there are times when the patient gets worse, sometimes following a fit or TIA, and then times when the patient seems a bit better and remains well for a while before the next episode.

Alzheimer-type and multi-infarct dementia can occur in the same patient so that there may be no clear distinction between the two types either during life or in the brain changes found after death.

Depression and dementia

Many older people develop depressive illnesses for which there are no apparent causes in their external lives. It can be difficult to distinguish between such an illness and the onset of dementia. Sometimes, during a depressive illness, a person can become confused and very forgetful but these clear up when the depression gets better with treatment. If there is doubt about the diagnosis, it is usual to treat the sickness as depression until there is more evidence that it is dementia.

Other types of dementia

About 10 per cent of cases of dementia in old age have a treatable cause and this is the main reason for investigations to be done. Acute illnesses, with a high temperature, can cause a state which looks like dementia, but when the underlying illness is treated with the appropriate antibiotic, the mind clears. Kidney failure, vitamin B12 deficiency and thyroid deficiency can also look like dementia and again respond to the appropriate treatment. Long-standing syphilis, brain tumours and AIDS can also look like dementia.

Huntington's disease and Pick's disease are genetic forms of dementia, and at the time of writing there is publicity about a rare form called Creutzfeld-Jakob disease and its possible connection with bovine spongiform encephalitis, also called BSE or mad cow disease.

Making the diagnosis. Is it important?

I have described the confusion surrounding John and the difficulties stemming from a lack of knowledge. Early in John's dementia, I knew in my heart that although something was changing in him it was not a clear-cut sickness. The doctor he saw at his medical check each year recognised his deterioration, but his general practitioner did nothing because there was no treatment to offer. And as far as the patient was concerned, the doctor was correct; it is possible that he was ill-informed of the facts and fearful of getting involved. A survey done by the Alzheimer's Disease Society found that over two-thirds of the doctors who replied thought that their training had been inadequate in the management of dementia. Two thousand carers replied to a questionnaire; 25 per cent of them felt that their doctor had inadequate knowledge and 60 per cent said that their doctor had not done a memory test on the patient. More than a third of the patients were not referred for a consultant opinion. A general view from the doctors was that early referral of the patient was not helpful but, on the other hand, they felt inadequate to offer any constructive help.

We like to believe that we live in enlightened times, and there is no shame about having a mental illness. But age-old prejudice takes a long time to change. Dementia is not treatable, the stigma of madness is attached to it and removal to a mental hospital is one of the spectres that looms.

Old people do become forgetful and it is difficult to know when normal forgetfulness ends and abnormal forgetfulness begins. Forgetfulness can become 'abnormal' if an old person starts to wander off in the night and the police have to bring him home, as happened with John. Or when he disappears while the family or a group of friends is on holiday, and then seems surprised that anybody should be alarmed. In addition to the failing memory, these are examples of the dementing person's loss of relationship with those around him.

Many people with dementia forget where they have put money, other valuables or clothes, and then accuse others of having taken them. It is common with increasing age to forget where you put your spectacles, and not too difficult to think that somebody else must have picked them up accidentally and put them somewhere else. However, in dementia, there is no longer any doubt in the patient's mind that somebody else has removed the missing objects, not accidentally but deliberately. While listening to narratives about those who have demented, I have noticed that the things that go missing often have a particular meaning for the patients. I write more about this in Chapter 9.

This sort of problem will probably not have a clear beginning, either because the patient has been naturally a little forgetful or because he has tended to lay responsibility for his actions at somebody else's door. He may, like John, always have been a bit of a miser and then become deluded about the amount of money he has. From there it is not a long step to delusions of poverty. 'I can no longer afford to buy food because I have no money' can become 'I can no longer afford to buy any food because my family has stolen all my money'. It causes immense distress to a family who find themselves unable to understand, or to defend themselves against, the false accusations of an apparently healthy member. The insidious onset makes recognition of the disease very difficult. The mixture of shame, loyalty and confusion can be very destructive for the carers, particularly if the nearest carer is the partner.

Although the general practitioner may be unable to do very much to help at this stage, recognition of the dementia can help carers to accept the changes, and the GP can provide them with an informed and listening ear. However, in one sense, the diagnosis is unimportant because there is no known way of taking the disease away, of making it better.

When I look for the meaning of the word 'diagnosis' in the *Dictionary of Word Origins*, I find 'the underlying meaning of Greek diagnosis was "knowing apart". It was derived from *diagignoskein* "distinguish, discern", a compound verb from the prefix *dia* "apart" and *gignoskein* "know, perceive" (a relative of English know). In post-classical times the general notion of "distinguishing" or "discerning" was applied specifically to medical examination in order to determine the nature of a disease.' I find that the importance of making a diagnosis is answered in this entry; the value of the discernment is for the carer and not for the patient.

Loss of recent memory occurs early in the disease and this failure accounts for many of the problems. The old man, or more commonly the old woman, will not remember the things that have occurred during the past week, day or even hours or minutes. This failure makes a conversation difficult because it is impossible for the patient to remember what somebody else has just said. She will find it easier to dominate the conversation and talk about the things she can remember, such as her childhood, her parents and early friends. If a doctor or nurse takes over and insists on answers to such questions as the day of the week, the old person may get very angry because these questions expose her confused mind. The loss of recent memory can lead to hazardous situations. For example, the old person may turn the gas taps on but her memory flips somewhere else before the gas is lit. As memory deteriorates, skills such as reading, writing, telling the time, knowing how to use the telephone or write a cheque go.

The dementing person may have a 'lost' look like a child's unsureness when he has strayed into an unfamiliar world, a look of bewilderment or of being haunted. If the inner sense of self is changing drastically there is likely to be a constant search for some sort of reassurance and support in the world around.

Early in the disease the dementing person forgets or confuses common words and uses unfamiliar ways to express common actions. My husband said that he must go to the other section (room) to cut the hair on his face (shave). Late in the disease, all intelligible speech may go and there will be incoherent mumbling and disjointed words.

There is general stiffening of muscles and difficulty in carrying out complicated movements. The gait is stiff and can look puppet-like. Late in the disease, the patient walks with small, stiff steps called *marche à petit pas*. Complicated movements, such as feeding and getting dressed, become difficult and then impossible even with help.

However well informed the doctor and the carers, the initial diagnosis is often made at a moment of crisis, when there is a clear need for outside help. The problems may have existed for a long time, without causing distress to the patient, until there is an outside demand for some measure of competence on the part of the patient. For John, the moment came when he drove his car into another without observing the rules of the road. For the old person who is living alone, it might be the departure of supportive neighbours and their replacement by intolerant ones. An old person who has been deteriorating over many years may be known to the neighbours and the tradesmen as needing care and support. The milkman is often one of the most practical and sensitive of social workers! The relatives, particularly if they live at a distance, can long remain in ignorance, and so can the professional carers. There may be mutterings of 'Something ought to be done about this' and 'Fancy relatives doing nothing to help this poor old man', but it is only when, one morning, the milk has not been taken off the doorstep and anxiety multiplies, that it is apparent that the ultimate responsibility does not lie with the milkman or the neighbours.

Occasionally, the apparent paranoia of the dementing person precipitates the crisis. He may make accusations of theft. Perhaps the bills are not paid, or the milkman cannot get his money and is told that relatives have stolen it. Again, a sudden decision has to be made to do something, and quickly.

Unacceptable behaviour can also precipitate the crisis. One woman coped heroically with her dementing mother in her small flat until the old lady became more confused during the night, and repeatedly mistook the laundry basket for the toilet. Suddenly the whole situation was no longer tolerable and her mother was sent to a psychogeriatric hospital. Another old lady was managing adequately in an ordinary old people's home until she decided to go for walks outside during the night, with nothing on. The home could cope with the wandering but not with the nakedness. In both these instances the crisis was precipitated not by a sudden deterioration in the patient's illness but the overstepping of a social limit for the carers.

If the nearest carer can be honest about her own needs and speak to the general practitioner, health visitor or practice nurse, in confidence, about the problems, such a crisis may be prevented. But this is only really helpful if the professional approached knows all the sources of help.

The general practitioner is in a key position and, if he is well informed and works in a team with a practice nurse, health visitor and possible a trained mental nurse, is well placed to make an early diagnosis and offer appropriate help and support. The GP, if he or the family feels it to be necessary, can arrange a home visit by a psychiatrist, geriatrician or psychogeriatrician. The exact title of the consultant is not as important as his or her interest in the problems associated with dementia. The 'expert' diagnosis of dementia is seldom as important as the wisdom of the professional in arranging the best support for the family and helping them to adjust to this tragic situation.

The assessment of the patient is best done at home, where the consultant physician, accompanied by the general practitioner, can see what the patient is like in his own 'patch'. They can also interview friends, relatives or other carers, and see for themselves what kinds of support may be needed. Further tests may be necessary to exclude treatable causes. For these, the patient may have to attend a hospital, preferably as an outpatient.

The debate about the extent of necessary investigations continues. There is no definitive diagnosis to confirm the presence of Alzheimer's disease during the lifetime of the patient. The most important tests are done to exclude the possibility of a treatable form of dementia. These may include blood tests, an electroencephalogram, a CT scan of the brain and x-rays. Other tests are done to establish the likelihood of Alzheimer's disease. The patient will have a general physical examination to exclude physical disease including anaemia. The blood pressure will be taken; a raised blood pressure with a history of 'passing out' at intervals may suggest multi-infarct dementia. There will be some assessment of sight and hearing. The physical examination will usually show some evidence of a patient's incontinence. An assessment will be made of the patient's mental state, in particular of the amount of loss of short-term memory.

After the investigations there should be an opportunity for the carer to meet the consultant and the general practitioner to discuss the next stages in the management of the patient. It is important for the carer to be honest about the size of the burden that she is able and willing to carry. This meeting is the opportunity to talk about day care, respite care or long-term residential care.

I stress that the diagnosis of Alzheimer's disease is of

greater importance for the carer than for the patient, once the possibility of a treatable type of dementia has been ruled out. The carer is the person best placed to decide what help is necessary, and she must try not to feel frightened, diffident or ashamed about putting her own needs at the top of the agenda. It is foolish, not heroic, to crack under the strain. Before the meeting to discuss the patient's management, the carer needs to ask herself some questions. It may be helpful to write them down. Am I well enough physically and mentally to go on coping? Can I go on coping with the patient living in the house with me? If he goes on living at home what help do I need now? Are there any special problems with which I should like help? Would it make a difference if he was away from me for one or more days a week? Would it help if I could be sure of two hours a day away from him?

Next on the agenda are the needs of the patient. What is best for the patient? Try asking the patient. It can all too easily be assumed that, because a patient is dementing, he no longer has any idea of what he wants. If he is asked where he wants to live he will usually say that he wants to stay at home. It is good to have a straightforward answer but this has to be balanced against the well-being of the carer. How much can she stand?

When somebody has started dementing there is an increased risk of accidents, particularly if he lives alone or spends any time alone. Some of the risks can and should be eliminated but it is not possible to remove all of them without confining the dementing person to bed in a locked room, which would, in any case, increase the risk of bronchopneumonia. The hazards include rugs on slippery floor surfaces, trailing flexes, unsafe electrical equipment, access to garden and household poisons and an unlocked medicine cupboard. Gas appliances will always be some risk, but modern gas stoves which light automatically are safer than those which must be lit with a match. All life is risky and it certainly cannot be made less so for the dementing person. An occupational therapist can assess the patient's home and make suggestions about suitable aids and alterations to make it safer and easier for the patient.

Arguing with the patient is an exhausting, frustrating and fruitless occupation. There are moments when it is better to assume that you and the patient are speaking different languages without an interpreter. It can then be easier to accept the different ways in which you and the patient view the world and each other, without the need for entanglement and further distress. One type of therapeutic management, called reality orientation, is designed to stimulate the patient's failing mental ability. The carer is advised never to agree with the patient if what the patient says is wrong. I think this may be more practical if the nearest carer is not somebody with emotional ties. A patient is more able to accept such direction in a nursing home or hospital than in his own home. The theory is good and the intention is to help the patient get on with his ordinary life, in the best way, with the minimum of fuss. He can then live in as socially acceptable a way as possible despite all his faculties failing. You must accept the reality that this is indeed second childhood for the patient but growing down, not growing up.

Communication and instruction should be kept to a minimum and never be confusing. One large clock showing the correct time and simple instructions in large print, perhaps with illustrations, about the way to the toilet and where to turn lights on and off can be helpful.

Establishing a support system

Making a support system work is like getting scaffolding up and secured. There will probably be a health visitor attached to your general practice, She is a trained nurse who has a specialist qualification in health visiting. Her experience is geared to preventive care. She will be a good source of information, counsel and support and will be able to put you in touch with other statutory services including social workers, occupational therapists, Meals on Wheels, the incontinence laundry service and the district nurses. She will also give you information about the local voluntary services, including the Alzheimer's Disease Society, Age Concern and Help the Aged. She will know about the local availability of day centres, respite care and residential care.

If a dementing person is living on his own, the more regular help he has, the better it will be for him. Visitors who arrive regularly, with a clear reason and for an obvious benefit, help him keep in touch with the day of the week and time of day, as well as providing him with necessary food, services and companionship. Neighbours are likely to remain more supportive if the whole burden of care does not fall on them.

Depending on the area of the country, there are different and changing arrangements about home care assistance. It will be necessary to find out what is available and then make the appropriate arrangements.

What about drugs?

Although much research work is being done on drugs which

could delay or relieve the mental deterioration in Alzheimer's disease, there is still no effective drug available at the time of writing this book. The monthly newsletter from the Alzheimer's Disease Society gives excellent updates on the state of current research.

Drugs can be used to control symptoms including constipation, sleeplessness, aggressive behaviour and severe agitation. This is an area where competent medical advice can be of enormous value.

Useful gadgets

An identity disc, engraved with the patient's name and telephone number, worn around the wrist, is valuable for the patient who tends to wander. Sometimes special door locks are fitted that the patient is unable to open, but this can cause much distress. If the patient can still be left alone for long periods he could have an aid call alarm; but he will need careful instruction in its use.

The Alzheimer's Disease Society

Any carer should join the society and possibly one of its local support groups. Some people will welcome the activities of such a group and be helped through the difficulties, while others may prefer to remain more isolated. The society produces a monthly newsletter and regularly updated information leaflets about benefits and resources.

Self-help groups

A self-help group can be a source of help for a carer, but the word 'carer' includes a multitude of individual and unique persons. No two carers will be alike, and that must never be forgotten. We must only cope and care to the limits of our own abilities and we must not seek to emulate anybody else. Much, too much, in our contemporary world is competitive, comparative and potentially destructive for the individual. 'If she can cope with all that work and worry, why can't I?' can get transposed into 'If I can't cope with that much and she can, then I am not of much use'.

All carers run the risk of overextending themselves and ending up as depleted of personhood as the dementing person they are caring for. Observing another's needs and ignoring one's own are commendable in the short term, but lead to intolerable and self-destroying stress in the longer term. Paradoxically, some carers do need to go on coping. A strong man caring for his wife with dementia may discover, within himself, hidden gifts of tenderness which he can now use to good effect. Perhaps for the first occasion in his life he can not only cry, but cry in public, and those watching him will think him a courageous man and not somebody to be despised. Even more important, he will not have contempt for the inner, feeling part of himself. He has discovered a hidden, almost lost talent. In a strange way, caring for his wife will give him a greater richness in his own life.

Legal aspects of dementia

A dementing person becomes forgetful and disorganised. He

may not have made a will; he probably will not know how much money he has or where it is. John had a habit of keeping small amounts of money in many different countries of the world. By the time he died he was out of touch with such things. The lost bits of money became part of the disintegration. The ability to manage day-to-day and more long-term financial affairs will not go all at once, but dissolve slowly. The progressive deterioration must be anticipated and plans made accordingly. This is not a morbid activity but an essential one for the well-being of the patient and possibly the spouse. Clear thinking, good professional advice and determined action save many painful situations before and after the patient's death.

Again these are facts which help to find a clearer path through the chaos, and to lay sure foundations for the carer's survival. It is important that the patient makes a will and that the closest carer knows where it is. Even if you are the spouse, you may not know if the dementing patient has made a will or where it is kept. This is particularly likely if the patient always tended to be secretive about money. The patient must, in the eyes of the law, be of 'testamentary capacity' in order to make a valid will. If he does not realise that he is making a will, and is not aware of the amount and nature of the property at his disposal, nor of his relationship with those to whom he is expected to leave it, he is no longer in a fit mental state to be making a will.

If the patient is no longer of testamentary capacity, a solicitor will be able to advise you. If, during the course of his dementia, the patient has made a will which is not believed to have been in accordance with his judgement before he deteriorated, it is possible to have it changed after his death with the agreement of the main beneficiaries of the will, by a Deed of Variation. However, this is not a simple option because Alzheimer's disease has an insidious onset and it is difficult to know at what point the patient lost his testamentary capacity. To rewrite a will after the death of a demented patient, when all those nearest are in the early stages of bereavement, is an emotional minefield. This option must be avoided if at all possible.

The Court of Protection, a part of the High Court in the UK, has the legal power to manage the affairs of those who, because of mental illness, including Alzheimer's disease, are not able to manage their own affairs. The Court needs medical evidence of this, and it then has the power to take over the patient's property and financial affairs and can appoint somebody with enduring power of attorney and/or a receiver.

An ordinary power of attorney can be made at any time for a person who is in his right mind and signs the appropriate forms. A person who is dementing but still able to manage his own affairs can also sign a power of attorney. This is a legal document which gives broad authority or limited powers to somebody of the patient's choosing to look after his affairs. It does not need to become fully operational until the mental state of the patient warrants it. It is a valuable procedure because the patient has the right to choose the person who will handle his affairs when necessary. One advantage is that there need be no delay in having access to the patient's financial resources if it should be necessary to sell a house or find money to pay nursing home fees

An enduring power of attorney is necessary when a person is no longer mentally able to manage his affairs. If a patient has not appointed anybody to have the power of attorney, the Court of Protection can appoint somebody as receiver. That person is then responsible for the management of the patient's money and property, under the control of the Court of Protection. I was the receiver for my husband and I had a named contact at the Court of Protection to whom I was responsible. If the patient's affairs have been taken over by the Court of Protection it can be asked that the will be found and deposited with the Court. The receiver can then have access to it, and any rewriting of it referred to the Court. If the patient has not made a will, the Court of Protection can be asked to do it before the patient's death.

You must inform the Driver and Vehicle Licensing Authority in the UK of any medically diagnosed condition (including Alzheimer's disease) which affects fitness to drive and will last for more than three months. The holder of the licence, not his doctor, is responsible for doing this and failure to do so invalidates his driving insurance.

What do patients with Alzheimer's disease die from?

I have heard Alzheimer's disease described as a 'slow goodbye' or an 'ongoing bereavement' or 'the empty house syndrome'. These all describe the long-lasting pain of watching somebody you once knew change and disintegrate. It is inappropriate to grieve or mourn while the person is physically still there, but it is appropriate to mourn for the spirit of the person that seems to have disappeared. One woman said, 'She is not really my mum because the mum I knew has died.' Another woman said, 'I married for better or for worse but this is not the person I married so am I still tied by my marriage vows?' The length of time of this ongoing bereavement will affect the time that the carer will need to recover after the death of the patient.

The disease can go on for so many years that the death of the body, as opposed to the death of the mind and spirit which has already, to a large extent, occurred, always seems a long way distant. In fact, life expectancy in Alzheimer's disease is always shortened and the end, when it does come, can be surprisingly rapid. Loss of weight nearly always occurs late in the disease, and in the last months wasting of the body may be rapid and profound. A patient is more likely to get ill if he is weak and unsteady. Because he is less active and remains seated in a chair or lying in a bed for long periods of time, he is more likely to get a chest infection followed by bronchopneumonia. Bronchopneumonia is a very merciful and peaceful end, but it may be necessary to say to the doctor in charge that you do not want antibiotics to be given. Ultimately the doctor's decisions must be made in the best interests of the patient; in this instance a doctor will usually listen to the nearest relative.

Most people, if they could state a preference, would, I believe, prefer to die in their own bed at home. Dementia does not necessarily exclude this possibility. Death is a normal process and one best completed within the home of the patient. Of course, if the patient is already in residential care, he will normally stay there. The process of dying is less familiar to most individuals now than it was a hundred years ago. Fewer children die, and so most of us have not experienced death at close quarters until our parents die. More deaths at an earlier age occur in a hospital or hospice with experts in charge. It is easy to assume that dying needs some sort of professional care. As a doctor, I had seen many people who were going to die and many dead bodies, but I had never shared anybody's death until I shared John's. I feel that it is good and right that the nearest relative should be there during dying. It is a lonely journey and the dying person needs the companionship of the person who has been closest to him emotionally.

If special help, such as pain relief, is needed, a doctor can be called. A district nurse will be available for any nursing help such as bathing, turning or changing the bed. You can be the person who is there to comfort, give sips of drink or moisten the mouth when necessary. You should, if possible, have somebody else available so that you can be looked after and fed and be able to take a rest.

If you or the patient is a practising religious person, you may well have been in touch with a priest or other religious leader and will have had an opportunity to talk about death and dying. You will have been able to ask him or your doctor about a good funeral director. It is not morbid to think and talk about this in advance. You may well feel less apprehensive about the inevitable death after you have considered the practical arrangements. When the death occurs you contact your doctor and then the funeral director who will guide you through the formalities and can be a competent and compassionate counsellor.

It can be beneficial for the family and close friends to see the body after it has been laid out because the person can look peaceful, younger and more like the person he was once before the onset of dementia.

The funeral is an important occasion for you and relatives and friends, whatever your religious beliefs and those of the patient. What sort of ceremony would he have liked if he could have discussed it with you before the onset of his disease? Thinking about the right ceremony to mark the end of his life can also be a start to mark the next stage of your own. Registration of the death and cremation or burial of the body are obligatory, but beyond those formalities are many options. If it is at all possible those closest to you and the patient should eat and drink together after the funeral. It need not be an elaborate meal.

Would he like flowers and music, a church service or one in the crematorium? Where would he have liked his ashes to be put if cremated? Perhaps there is a place to commemorate your happiest times together. These decisions can be stepping-stones along your own road to recovery and re-integration.

Bereavement

With Alzheimer's disease, bereavement has started long before the death of the patient. It may have gone on for as long as ten years during his lifetime. Dementia, being a dis-integration of the whole person, can be felt by those closest to the patient as a threat to their own integrity. Denial of some of the feelings aroused while caring for a dementing person is normal and necessary, but at some point the carer needs to look at the shut-away feelings in order to make a full recovery. Recovery after a death from Alzheimer's disease can take a very long time because of the nature of this long-lasting death.

There have been many descriptions of the stages of grief. Elizabeth Kubler-Ross, in 1970, described them as denial, anger, bargaining, depression and acceptance. They have since been described as alarm, searching, mitigation, anger, guilt and finally gaining a new identity. They have also been described as shock and disbelief, developing awareness and resolution.

These descriptions may be useful for the bereaved person and help her see her feelings as normal, acceptable and understood. So-called stages along the way help to give a sense that somebody else has been this way before. But they are unhelpful if they provide a check list of normality. If the bereaved person feels that her grief is not completed during the 'normal' time of a year, there can be self-imposed pressures. 'I should try harder and make more effort' or 'I ought to have accepted it by now.' Bereavement can become another disease to be handed over to a doctor for diagnosis and treatment and then become somebody else's responsibility. The bereaved person needs to experience the loss and take responsibility for her future. Bereavement is as unique and individual as the number of people going through it. It is a lonely experience, an echo of what birth was and death will be.

All the 'should' ideas can be intellectually understandable but emotionally barren. It is easy to get caught up in the 'shoulds' and 'oughts' which can only perpetuate the vicious circle of confusion, anger and despair. The *Shorter Oxford English Dictionary* defines bereavement as 'deprive, rob, strip, dispossess of'. This definition emphasises the passivity of what has happened. It is something over which you had no control. I think that sense of being a receiver can help to resolve and clarifiy the feelings of meaninglessness.

In one study of thirty-five people who had a breakdown after bereavement, it was found that there were two common factors. One was a tendency for the grief to have been prolonged; and the other was for the reaction to bereavement to have been delayed. Bereavement after Alzheimer's disease must always incorporate these two risk factors. In the group of those who had broken down there was preoccupation with ideas of guilt and self-reproach.

In prolonged and unresolvable grief, all the previous experiences of loss in that person's life, possibly back to early childhood, may be reawakened. I felt at one point that my own sense of loss had gone on for so long that full recovery would be impossible. Endurance of the last of my own days was all that I could reasonably expect. Every loss, from infancy on, can be stirred and erupt, and the pain can become so great that it must be avoided and denied. The disintegration and death of a near person strikes chords that sing out our own lack of integrity. Each stage in the disintegration of the patient throws out another wave of terror for the carer. These shock waves of pain can cause disabling distress if acknowledged during the patient's life; but at a later date their recognition and acceptance can be the start of a new and deeper understanding of the self. There can then be a remarkable opportunity, not only for eventual recovery from all the bereavements, but also for a new vision of the way in which the carer can live the rest of her own life.

A spouse, particularly a wife, may cling to the relationship because there is a loss of status in widowhood. To cling to a relationship in which the meaning is lost can prevent facing up to the living of life as a single person. Denial of feelings can become a way of life and a strategy for survival. The anger and sense of outrage about the continual 'robbery' of Alzheimer's, which can appear to have no limits, become inadmissible. Anger as a stage in bereavement is 'normal'; but this state may already have continued for many years in the chronic death from Alzheimer's disease. The carer has not been robbed, rejected or abandoned once by the death of the patient, but repeatedly, as the patient removed himself from her and the relationship during his long disintegration. Ongoing and self-destructive anger can find a temporary escape route as depression or a physical illness, but these conditions do not resolve stresses within the carer.

Long-standing denial of angry feelings and intense emotional pain can cause a sense of 'I will not ever feel too much again. If I felt too much about anything it might hurt and I could not bear it. It might destroy me utterly.' These unspoken, even unrecognised thoughts can be a way of avoiding intense pain but they also keep out experiences of joy and peace. It may appear safer, but it is a sad and inadequate way of readjustment and a constantly self-inflicted deprivation, though not a conscious one. My hunch is that this same sequence of events occurred during early life to the patient who develops Alzheimer's disease, and I shall write more about this in the last two chapters of the book.

One of the unexpected benefits of the American renaming of all cases of senile dementia as Alzheimer's disease in 1975 is the lessening of the terror of the disease. Once named, there is the assumption that it can be identified and dealt with. The strange noise that wakes you in the night is infinitely more bearable when it can be identified as the rats in the roof. A telephone call to the rodent operator and 'treatment' of the rats will restore quiet to the night hours. But giving a name without evidence to support it can only provide temporary amelioration and then the quest must be abandoned or continued into unknown territory, which is frightening. Truth and reality are not comfortable options.

Alzheimer's disease is known to be a disease that is not preventable or curable. It runs its course, the patient dies and these facts can be reasonably distanced from feelings of guilt and desolation. Some of the distress can then be shifted into reading books about bereavement, and pressing for more research into the scientific nature of the disease and search for a cure. Recovery from bereavement has more to do with experiencing all the losses with heart and guts than knowing them with the intellect and in the head. That is the way of disintegration and not of reintegration. A daughter whose mother demented said that her mother's whole life was in her head, and when the mother lost her marbles, her whole world fell to pieces. It is only through becoming open to the pain at every level, and then daring to stick with it, that solid and lasting recovery can occur. The most valuable helpers are those who can stay alongside in your grief and do not always want you to cheer up and deny the misery. There does come a time when a degree of stoicism can also be important.

The connection between the acceptance of the pain and resolution of grief is beautifully expressed in *The Prophet* by Kahlil Gibran.

And a woman spoke, saying, Tell us of Pain.

And he said:

Your pain is the breaking of the shell that encloses your understanding.

Even as the stone of the fruit must break, that its heart may stand in the sun, so must you know pain.

And could you keep your heart in wonder at the daily miracles of your life, your pain would not seem less wondrous than your joy;

And you would accept the seasons of your heart, even as you have always accepted the seasons that pass over your fields.

And you would watch with serenity through the winters of your grief.

Much of your pain is self-chosen.

It is the bitter potion by which the physician within you heals your sick self.

Therefore trust the physician, and drink his remedy in silence and tranquillity:

For his hand though heavy and hard, is guided by the tender hand of the Unseen.

And the cup he brings, though it burn your lips, has been fashioned of the clay which the Potter has moistened with his own sacred tears.

CHAPTER 3

More steps in my quest

I have looked at John's life, written it and made an attempt
to understand it and to disentangle the story of his life from
the story of my own. I have attempted to grasp the present
state of scientific and medical knowledge about the disease
and looked at current ways of treating and managing patients
with the condition. However, at this stage of my quest, I
realised that I had little understanding about Alzheimer's
disease; the more I knew about what had happened the more
I wanted to understand why it happened. I looked again and
harder at John, and at the disease, and wondered if John had
been more or less all right before the disease attacked him;
or was it something different from ordinary illnesses, with a
mysterious and much deeper level of meaning. My feelings
that it was something different were increased each time
somebody spoke to me about their friend or relative who
had the condition, or who had died from it; and I began to
see strange small similarities in the life stories.

The choice of words

At some moments it is correct for me to write 'he' or 'she'
but at other times the person I refer to could be either male
or female, and at those times I have chosen to write 'he' in
the original German and Old English sense of 'human being,

person' and therefore it does not denote specifically a male, but a member of humankind.

I also use the words 'story' and 'narrative' repeatedly. Here I do not mean something that has been invented or is in any way untrue or a fabrication. I use the words to distinguish the account of a narrator from a medical case history, which is designed and structured by the questioner to elicit information from which to make a diagnosis. I needed a discipline, but not control or a planned structure for each encounter.

Allowing interviews to happen in this way has given me quite different information from anything I could have imagined at the beginning. Initially I thought that I should be writing as a medical journalist, up to a point dictating the ideas on the page in the same way as the writer of a mystery thriller, who knows the final outcome and remains in charge. How foolish of me to have said at one moment that I wished to search with unprejudiced eyes and ears, and at the same time to have expected to be in charge of the writing. On the way I have had many surprises. I know that the finish of this book will be the start of another voyage of discovery because, like a poem or a painting, it can never be finished, only abandoned.

I have used the word 'patient' on many occasions because it has been the simplest way of identifying the person who has Alzheimer's disease.

Familiar themes

One of the first similarities I marked were the missing parents. I looked at John's life story and saw again his family tree. John's father, Robin, grew up without a mother from the age of two. He was sent from India to the UK at the age of eight for his education and, from then for a number of years, he was without both his father and his mother. I know very little of his story and have no knowledge of any parent substitutes that he found. John's father and mother separated when John was ten and he was brought up by his mother and three of her sisters. By the time that his parents were reunited, John had already started work. He, therefore, grew up through later childhood and adolescence without a father, in a strongly female household. When I listened to other stories, I began to hear echoes of this theme of a missing parent, more often a father, or a lack of a strong male influence. The pattern of the missing or weak father might be repeated in an absentee, weak or deserting husband.

Another theme that ran through the narratives was missing babies. John was an only child. I understood from his mother, who was one of eight children, that his birth had been very difficult but I know nothing else. She was already an old and frail lady when I first met her. I believe that she would have liked other children but I do not know whether she had lost any. Four years passed between her marriage and John's birth. When I listened to other narratives I heard echoes of the missing baby theme, either deaths of small children near to the person who subsequently developed Alzheimer's disease, or stillbirths, or miscarriages. I have been aware of the shadow of a dead baby over the person who dements. I saw in John's life an early isolation and I have seen that theme repeated.

A third theme which was common was a search, in adult life, for a home. This need was so strong that it seemed to reflect an earlier period in life, when the child felt homeless and unrooted. John desperately wanted a home, a place that was special for him in which to live his old age. He needed to know that he belonged. He had been uprooted when he was ten and lived the next years in other people's homes. He had travelled the world for most of his life and had seldom known a place that he felt was home. I write, later in this book, about roots and being uprooted. One of John's dreams was to buy land in Scotland and plant trees. We acted out his quest for his true home when we moved to Caithness. For many reasons he did not find roots in either his outer world or his inner understanding of this desperate search for a true home.

A further theme was the importance of cars. John always wanted to have his own car and would have found it difficult either to share a car or relinquish control. He went on driving until late in his disintegration, when he caused a road accident. At that point he lost control because of police action. I have heard this theme repeated in the narrations I have looked at in detail, and also in many passing observations. One woman who had been diagnosed as having Alzheimer's disease rented a car and had not driven it more than fifty miles when she drove into a wall and the car was written off. Later she drove through red lights in a city centre, refused to stop and was arrested by the police. She was normally a law-abiding citizen. There have been other accounts of careless and uncharacteristic driving which, looked at in retrospect, seem to have been one of the earliest signs of the onset of disintegration.

Yet another common theme has been the confusing of key people, late in the dementia. I looked at the patient in the final state of dependency, and then at the key person to whom he would still turn for help, and might recognise. I wondered if this person represented consistently the strongest anchor figure at a very early stage in the patient's life. On one occasion, during the last days of John's life, when he was in bed with bronchopneumonia, he surprised a nurse by getting out of bed, going to his chest of drawers, on which were two photographs, and taking one of them back to bed with him. One of the photographs was of his mother and the other of me. When I was told of this incident I very much wanted to know which he had chosen but the nurse did not remember. I now see that the choice was irrelevant, because I represented his mother, the strong woman and the old anchor in his life. While I listened to narrations I detected this important figure who appeared early in life, was often discarded later in childhood but late, in the disintegration, was replaced by somebody who represented that original key figure.

For each patient who had been in a threatened position in early childhood, there was a strong need to cling to some particular sort of 'specialness'. This mark of being exceptional had to be possessed through their entire life; and the individual hung onto it at the expense of everything else. The need for specialness included many ordinary things, such as having a husband or wife, a large house, plenty of money and a secure place in society, but these could become so important that they defined the value of the person. These external values make the owner vulnerable, because at any time they could be split off by ill health, bereavement or poverty and then the protection of these outer values is shed.

These common themes, a missing or dead baby, a missing parent, an unstable sense of home or unrootedness, suggest that each of these people had known insecurity early in life. If a child has experienced terrifying insecurity it is normal that he should seek to find his own security and to keep control. It occured to me, however, that he might, at some point in life, be 'offered' a more creative and fulfilling life but he might not dare to allow a chink in his rigid walls, to accept any degree of insecurity. He dare not, at any time, lose any control over his own security and over those around him. In this case the organisation would reign supreme at the price of creativity. I already knew that John did not want to know about his father's talents and had given his best paintings to a stranger. He had also put obstacles in the way of my writing and painting.

Problems and solutions

In orthodox medicine, there are problems that must be solved and there are well recognised methods of procedure. You take a case history from the patient, make a diagnosis with the help of suitable diagnostic tests and then prescribe the appropriate treatment with the object of a cure. It was a shock to realise that in the way I was searching there might not be any answers. I realised that the most I could achieve at present was to see more clearly. I had to start without preconceived ideas, look, look and look again and then set out in words, if possible, what I saw. I then had to be content for others to see more, from different perspectives. All I could do was suggest a new and different angle for the looking. I described it to myself as looking into an enormous multi-faceted crystal. I knew that there was the truth at the centre of the crystal. Most people were looking in at one angle and seeing one aspect of the truth. I wanted to go a little distance away and look from another angle. What they saw and what

I saw would all be part of the truth but from different perspectives. I knew that I would not come up with new answers, let alone THE answer. I also knew this was an uncomfortable, vulnerable and isolated position, out of step with current trends.

I made a commitment to see with unprejudiced eyes and hear with open ears as far as possible. In other words, I was not to look at the narratives in the way a doctor examines a specimen. I must attempt to describe what I see and my own conclusions without the use of special words, either medical, religious or psychological. Words that are in any way 'special' to these disciplines can act as shortcuts for the initiated but as stumbling blocks for those who are not in that position. Special words can close doorways to understanding while simple words open them. There are moments when I wish I were an expert, a neurologist, a psychiatrist, a theologian, psychologist or a philosopher, but I am none of these. In orthodox medicine, if there is not a recognised solution to an identified problem, it is a matter of considerable concern. Some strategy will be set up for the necessary research. It is assumed that every problem known to man will be capable of solution with sufficient money and the exercise of man's intellect and scientific equipment.

Death falls outside the possibility of medical cure and there are some diseases, including Alzheimer's, which are not yielding up their secrets to the scientific method yet. We may have to see them and understand them in a different way. Do we have to knock down the walls of scientific thought and be prepared to go through some sort of emptiness without the crutches of the intellect? Perish the idea! I remember arithmetic textbooks in my school days, with the correct answers at the back of the book. But supposing the problems were pictures, not figures, and at the back of the book there were no correct answers. There might be a palette of colours for altering or developing the pictures and making fresh images.

It is a strange thought that the intellect could run up against the buffers and fail to produce the solution, a sort of sterility. For the micropathologist, there is progress in the understanding of Alzheimer's disease and for the neurophysicist and the neurochemist and for many other men of science. But so far these intellectual and scientific concepts have not helped me to understand how I may live my own old age so that I do not disintegrate.

Leaving a space

And so my quest jumped from the relatively safe world of scientific research and ordered, rational, intellectual understanding into a very different world of hunches, intuitions and uncertainties, a search for the possible meanings of the common themes that haunt the narratives.

I have been guided and encouraged by Peter Brook's words in *There Are No Secrets*. He is writing about directing plays but I believe that his ideas also apply to any creative activity, including the living of a whole life or any small part of a life. For me, at this time, it means the encouragement to go on with the search through many times of doubt and confusion. 'The director must have from the start what I have called a "formless hunch" that is to say a certain powerful but shadowy intuition that indicates the basic shape, the source from which the play is calling him. Day after day, as he intervenes, makes mistakes or watches what is happening on the surface, inside he must be listening, listening to the secret movements of the hidden process.'

I have become aware, as I have listened to each narrative, of the inner drama of each of the patients. Towards the end of life, the drama must either come together for the final act of death at the last curtain, or, in a meaningless way, be dispersed, fragmented and confused with all the peripheral players. I have been aware of both the outer and visible stage of each actor/patient and of that inner and invisible stage.

Peter Brook, in his essay 'The Slyness Of Boredom' writes about actors leaving an inner space and of what may come out of it. 'This is hard for the Western mind to accept, having turned "ideas" and the mind into supreme deities for so many centuries. The only answer is in direct experience, and in the theatre one can taste the absolute reality of the extraordinary presence of emptiness, as compared with the poverty-stricken jumble in a head crammed with thinking.' And later he writes 'that if one doesn't search for security, true creativity fills the space. . . A true artist is always ready to make any number of sacrifices in order to reach a moment of creativity. The mediocre artist prefers not to take risks, which is why he is conventional. Everything that is conventional, everything that is mediocre is linked to this fear. The conventional actor puts a seal on his work, and sealing is a defensive act. To protect oneself, one "builds" and one "seals". To open oneself, one must knock down the walls. . . The true process of construction involves at the same time a sort of demolition. This means accepting fear. All demolitions create a dangerous space in which there are fewer crutches and fewer supports. . . One needs to do the preparation in order to discard it, to build in order to demolish.'

I do not think it fanciful to apply Peter Brook's words to

the living of every ordinary life. I have realised, as my own search has gone on, that each of my formless hunches has had to be exposed to reality. Some have been abandoned but others have come to life in surprising ways. I see that they only come alive if I dare to abandon any preconceived ideas. All certainty goes, trepidation arrives and trust is often in short supply. Certainty often means organisation, and total organisation is death to any creativity.

I know that half of my hunches will be wrong and must be abandoned; that is part of the demolition along the way. For example, at the start of my quest, I wondered, from the world distribution of Alzheimer's disease, if it were more common in people who had been brought up as Protestants than as Roman Catholics. That hunch did not stand up to hard looking.

Nature does not allow a vacuum and much work is necessary to keep emptiness in a space. A full diary, busy-ness and superlative organisation are the usual ingredients to fill any space in our present culture. If left empty, without any discipline at the boundaries, the space will be over-run with many invaders. There is a paradox between the discipline which is necessary to guard the boundaries of the space and allow a creative spark to develop, and the organisation which fills the space and exterminates any particle of creativity.

While I write this chapter I struggle against time because of the publisher's deadline. I also struggle with pain. A week ago I broke ribs on the right side of my chest after a fall down a steep and unlit step in a cathedral. The pain is severe and I am not able to walk far or drive a car but with enough painkillers I can manage to sit at my desk for several hours each day and work. Therefore my own space is bounded in one direction by time and in another direction by pain. I can either see this event as a problem that needs a solution or I can use it as an opportunity for understanding of a different kind. I shall look at it from the doctor's viewpoint first. I telephoned my general practitioner the morning after the fall because I was in pain. He asked me all the correct questions, heard my description of the grating of bony ends and the place of the bruise. He could hear over the telephone that I was not breathless and therefore could not have a punctured lung. I live in the country a long way from his surgery. There is an influenza epidemic at the moment, he is busy and I am not able to drive my car. There is no treatment for fractured ribs. Long ago, broken ribs were strapped to relieve the pain and the patient frequently got a chest infection because he could not breathe as deeply. The doctor offered me painkillers and I accepted. I did not need a visit and he did not offer one. I was content with the telephone consultation. His problem was solved and at one level so was mine. There was nothing to do but put up with the pain and wait for six weeks and the bones will heal.

At another level none of this did anything to solve what I see as my problem. I must finish a book. If I take enough painkillers to stop the pain my mind is clouded and I am not able to write. If I do not take any, the pain is too much of a distraction. I live alone, am not able to go shopping and cannot walk as far as the postbox. There is a multitude of small practical problems to which I must find solutions. I can see the injury as entirely nasty, negative and something that should never have happened. I might even think of suing the cathedral authorities for letting the public loose in unlit choir stalls.

However, out of this is coming something quite different.

When I stop looking for a solution to these problems of immobility and pain I begin to see another scenario. At this moment I need an honourable release from one or two obligations before Christmas so I can devote myself to writing without interruption. I now have complete seclusion in a warm, centrally heated cottage. I am sufficiently mobile to get to all the necessary parts of my home for the essential functions of living and writing. When I stop seeing this incident as either all black or all white I can see that it as an acceptable and welcome shade of grey.

At yet another level I can see a different and mysterious scenario. The break is on the right-hand side of my chest. In ancient wisdom the liver, which is on the right side of the abdomen underneath the ribs, is the seat of feeling and emotion. Now I have broken that firm barrier that protects my liver just at the time that I write about breaking the walls of intellectual certainty and daring to live in a state of uncertainty. My liver, the bodily and symbolic representation of my feelings, is vulnerable because the protective barrier of the rib-cage is damaged, and my feelings are raw while I struggle to understand the meaning of Alzheimer's disease. My head tells me that the fracture and the pain are wrong, a problem to be solved. But I am impotent and helpless. Another six weeks and the bones will be healed without any action or control on my part.

A medical friend reminded me that the pain would become less acute when the ruptured ends of the bones began to knit together. I think of his words and have a feeling of awe and wonder that an enormous army of invisible and minuscule knitters is busy night and day putting this interruption in my rib-cage together again. I have a sense of a miracle, one that happens to me and everybody alive, all the time. Bits of body are constantly being repaired and replaced and invaders repelled; but I had not seen it this way before now. Healing is a normal process provided we give it a chance.

Though I said that there is nothing I can do, I must keep everything very simple. I must try not to drop things on the floor because I am not able to pick them up, and I must live in an orderly fashion so that I do not waste energy looking for lost property. I must not work too long because I am easily fatigued. I must lie down at night even if I am not able to sleep, and remain aware of how much as well as how little I can do. My present space is clearly demarcated by the realities of time and space. Within those boundaries I have a particular job to complete. In a small way it is a like a miniature of any life. There is a job of work to do and perhaps each one of us has a particular job to do during life. There is no time or energy to spare for any complaint about the fairness of what has happened.

The knitting together is like the acceptance of the whole of ourselves, and the whole package that life has given us. The good and the bad are the raw materials from which the artist paints pictures and the potter makes bowls. The raw materials of life are a mixed lot but a gift is what is given and sometimes the packaging can be deceptive. The gift that ultimately becomes a blessing can be presented as a curse. Acceptance is the key. The gift arrives and you have the choice to accept or reject it. In fairy stories this is a normal and common phenomenon, as in the Sleeping Beauty and the wicked fairy. There has been a shift during the past two hundred years from seeing fairy stories as timeless wisdom for everybody, to seeing them as for children only, while the underlying truths are dismissed as irrelevant for adults.

Choosing the narrators

I decided that I would look at six stories of people who had Alzheimer's disease, three in the USA and three in the UK, of which John's story would be one. Although it was I who made the choice of the narrators, and either knew or knew about each of those people, I knew very little about the person who had demented. With one exception, I did not go back to any of the people who had contacted me after the publication of my first book on Alzheimer's disease. I wanted to discover more about the life of the person before he demented, rather than concentrate on detailed accounts of the disintegration after the condition became apparent.

I let my imagination wander around the people I knew who had demented and those near to them with whom I could speak. I began to have strong hunches about those whom I could ask to be narrators and those that, for one reason or another, I could not. I did not understand initially that these choices were an important step in my understanding of Alzheimer's disease. I began to make tentative lists of people I might ask and to look at the qualities I was seeking in the narrator. I also had to understand why there were people to whom I felt that it would not be right to make an approach, and the reasons for my reluctance.

The narrator had to be a relative, close friend or partner of the person who demented, so that they could tell me about the person's life and personality before and after the onset of the disease. She must be prepared to commit the time and energy to enter with me into this search. She must be articulate and open minded. I realised that it was very important that the narrator could be objective about the patient. I looked at the possible narrators and thought very hard about this question of objectivity. Did I mean that the patient must already be dead? Or live at a great geographical distance from the narrator? Should the narrator not be personally involved in the day-to-day care of the patient? Certainly death a few years earlier made it easier to see a broader perspective, as I knew with my own husband, but I came to see that it was not the only reason. I saw that the idea that Alzheimer's disease could have something to do with the person who had it could be too terrifying for people close to it, because it undermined the rational approach to disease. The threat of disintegration, if the potential narrator was genetically related to the patient, could only be kept at sufficient distance by believing the scientific view of disease. One group of potential narrators about whom I had doubts were rational people with strong opinions about disease. It would not be possible for them to look objectively and with clear eyes at any alternative ideas. On two counts I would not ask them; first, because it could not further my own understanding, and second, because it would be a threat to their own walled-up viewpoint.

One daughter who was willing to speak with me had, as she saw it, an idyllic relationship with her mother. I realised that this vision could not be objective. One man I could not ask because he felt badly threatened by his sister's dementia and was fearful about a genetic inheritance. It would have been intrusive on my part to ask something with so much potential for pain. I knew that both the blandness and fear were personal defence systems against something seen as too threatening. If it was considered as disease, separate from the person concerned, although there was still the fear of a genetic inheritance, it was easier to deny and keep walled-off, in the same way as the disease could be walled-off from the person who has it. This wicked disease struck, everything was fine until this happened, and if only there was a cure for the disease everything could be fine again. It is one defence, but a fragile one, and leaves no opportunity for any choice for the individual who does feel threatened.

I knew that there was another group of people that I could not ask to be narrators, for a different reason which I could not at first fathom. I allowed my imagination to roam around this scenario. If I try to see each person, not as some entity detached from other people, but as part of a related whole, what do I see in my mind's eye? I start to see people as more like trees in a forest. All the parts I can see are distinct; the leaves are of varied colour and separately identifiable. But what happens below ground? Of course my mind comes to roots and rootedness and the earth. What has any of this to do with Alzheimer's disease? Rootedness and finding roots has much to do with the idea of searching for a home and family and close connections at the outer level. I heard this refrain many times. In old age this search for the right home, the dream home, a quiet place to retire to, somewhere we were always so happy, is common.

When I go on with my reverie about roots, I begin to see more clearly why there are some people I can ask to speak about a relative who has demented and some that I cannot. I can ask those people, nearest the patient, whom I see as sturdy healthy trees, of a known and recognised species, with enough light and air around them. There are others that are not so sturdy and independent. There is a feeling that the tree which is breaking up may have roots that are intertwined with the person to whom I wish to speak or, if already dead, has fallen and left the survivor damaged, inadequately rooted, with their water and food supply threatened. I cannot speak to this person because it could provoke further damage to an already threatened survival at a deep and invisible level. At this stage in my search I must remember these images and wait to understand them better, or possibly discard them if they are of no help in my understanding.

Two of the people who were eventually narrators had difficulties in distinguishing their stories from those of the patients. Always the teller's story came back, not the story of the one I believed to be the key person. I began to wonder if the teller who cannot distinguish her story from the patient's does not know her story and therefore is not able to tell the patient's story as a distinct entity. Is this a further image of entangled roots?

One friend was ready and willing to be helpful and I always enjoy her company. She is articulate, literary and intelligent but my hunch said ' No'. I decided that it was because she is so totally intertwined with her mother's story that she cannot distinguish herself from it. Her mother is still alive and as she slips into a fantasy world, the daughter is in some ways following her. She now sees her mother's 'escapades' as very amusing. At one level they are, but at another level the disintegration of a human being is always tragic and this level of understanding is absent in the daughter. I believed that this entanglement in the fantasy would prevent any possibility of objectivity.

At the moment I am thinking about the narrators and not about the patients; but if I allow the walls of my medical training to fall down, or I take steps to aid the demolition, I see that all people have the potential for integration and for disintegration. At the same time I begin to demolish the walls between a person who has a disease and the disease itself. On one side of me are those whom I cannot ask because they are reasonable, rational and walled up and on the other the people whose roots are entangled. If I go back to the idea of an inner space, could it be that the rational ones have filled the space with organisation and walled it up, while the others have their roots so entangled that they have lost the boundaries of their own inner space?

Now I wonder if these opposite extremes are present in everybody, both those who disintegrate in old age and those who do not, and continue a process of coming together. Is this to do with an imbalance or balance between the opposites? Is there a way in which they are held together in those people who continue to integrate in their old age? What is it that keeps the balance between the impenetrable walls of extreme rationalism and a loss of the boundaries? Ironically most people who dement are either safely locked up in a home or are free but unsafely wandering everywhere and anywhere; but the choice between the one and the other is seldom, if ever, made by the patient.

The potential narrator who is not able to see the opposites in her relationship with the patient will not be able to give a balanced account. It is easier to slam the door on the bit that is opposite than go through the pain of allowing it in. Are the people who dement those who only see the good, the light, the rational view and who have become the 'too good' people? In one sense John was the 'too good' chairman. There are the 'too good' mothers, the 'too good' nuns and monks, the ones who succeed in their particular niche and have to hang on to it to have any worth. They have endlessly to justify their existence and prove their worth. They cannot let go of their values and acknowledge any other part of themselves, the weaker and darker bits that fail and forget, are black and helpless. In all these pictures I begin to see a common sense of a lack of feeling. It is as though control of the person's life is so important that feelings of sadness, joy, failure and loss are unacceptable. The core value of these people seems to be in their outer achievements.

I gradually whittled down the possible narrators to five and they all agreed to help me search. Of the six accounts, four of the people with Alzheimer's disease are dead. Of the two still alive, the narrator for one lives at a great distance and the other is a remarkably objective person, genetically unrelated to the patient.

Establishing the boundaries

Having agreed with the two narrators in the UK and the three in America, I needed to decide how and when we met. My hunch was that it would require two sessions. I use the word 'session' to define a clearly defined space in time and place in which the narrator and I gave ourselves totally to hearing and receiving the story of the patient. It was not possible to continue with this degree of concentration for more than two hours before a break was necessary. On most occasions, although two hours had been set aside, one and a half hours was sufficient to complete that part of the work together. By that time both the narrator and I were tired and needed a break. When I remained with the narrator during the break we observed a discipline of not speaking about the patient. I thought initially that the break should be at least twenty-four hours and not longer than a week. The forces of reality made me change this idea on two occasions. On one occasion, because of the sickness of the narrator, the interval between meetings was more than a week and on another occasion, because I travelled to the narrator, the two sessions took place in one day; but we had a break of three hours without speaking of the patient. It was possible, but tiring for both of us.

It was important to select the physical space with care. Two of the sessions were in a friend's house in America and they allowed me *carte blanche* to choose the room. Although the one I chose had five doors, one into a conservatory, it had a feeling of privacy and seclusion uninterrupted by sounds from beyond this space. I did not want to use a tape recorder for two reasons. The first was that I felt its presence and movement would be an intruder in the meeting; and the second was that playing back tapes would control my responses to the story that I had heard. I kept a notebook and pencil with me and could make brief notes without any sense of intrusion for myself or the narrator. I discussed this means of recording with the narrator.

On each occasion I had previously contacted the narrator by letter or telephone, with one exception when a close friend acted as intermediary. I sent a brief synopsis of the book I hoped to write, and at the first meeting I spoke about the book and the nature of my search. All the narrators knew that I am medically qualified and I explained the differences between what I was doing and the taking of a medical case history. They could all appreciate and respond to the difference. As far as possible, I listened to the account and did not ask questions.

I have changed all the names, and those I have chosen are acceptable to the narrators. I have changed places and circumstances in order to preserve anonymity but I have tried not to change anything that would imperil the essential truths of the narrative.

The choosing of the narrators and the establishment of the discipline of the meetings taught me a little more about the nature of Alzheimer's disease. Here I must reiterate that what I was learning and discovering was in no way an alternative to the scientific and orthodox medical knowledge which I had already studied but was an addition, a pushing out of my own boundaries of understanding.

CHAPTER 4

Amanda

During the first two-hour session with Amanda's daughter, Patsy, I was given a vivid picture of the landscape surrounding the central character, Amanda. But, in a most mysterious way, the central figure in the drama remained a blank space. It was as though I were watching an opera set with a crowded and brilliantly dressed chorus and well-defined supporting cast but the star performer in the centre was a white gap. Patsy and I had been sitting together in a tranquil wooden-frame house on a cliff overlooking a beautiful bay in Northern California. This was the first narrative I had heard in the way that I had decided was right for my search and I assumed that this was the way it would always be. At the end of two hours I knew almost nothing about the patient but a great deal about her family setting, her forebears and her descendants.

Patsy and I planned to do other things together for the next twenty-four hours and not speak about Amanda. There were many questions that I wanted to ask and lines of interest that I wanted to pursue, but I felt it was better for both of us to have a break occupied with walking and other shared interests before our next session together. I thought that in this second period of concentrated thought about Amanda I should be able to fill in the central character and watch and hear her come alive. However, this is not exactly what did happen.

After the two sessions with Patsy were completed, during the course of the next few days, I met, by coincidence, two other people of Patsy's generation who had known Amanda very well. I began to realise that I would only learn more about Amanda before her dementia by observing the pieces of her which she seemed to have implanted in the young people closely connected with her. Instead of seeing the whole picture as a positive print, I had to attempt to understand it as a negative, to see the spaces rather than the shapes. At moments then, and later, I had the feeling that Amanda was a creator of people. She had a profound influence on them and their whole lives; they saw her in terms of what she had done for them and to them. But I could find no answer to my search for what sort of person she was. It was as though she were a potter who had left her pots and disappeared without much trace of herself, a creator dissolved in her creation.

I began to have a picture in my mind of somebody investing all of herself outside herself, and never getting sufficient return from those investments to remain solvent. It was like listening to a story of progressive bankruptcy, not in terms of money, although that played a part, but in terms of something of a different value. I began to look at the symbolism of value, money, investment and a demand for return on the investment.

If I was to learn more about Amanda I had to look at and listen to the three people whom I met while I was in California and see the parts of her she had invested outside herself. This was at total variance from any sort of medical case history that I had ever taken or read. At the time I knew that I must keep the same discipline in my observations as I should keep if I were taking a medical history, but here

I must not ask questions to direct the narrative and I must allow my imagination and intuition freedom to see another dimension. It is almost as though the currencies were incompatible; there was no common currency or accepted rate of exchange.

Amanda's mother, Olga, was born in Scandinavia in 1880, was adopted, at the age of three, by Americans whom neither she nor her parents had met, and 'shipped' to New York. Very early in life she must have learned the way to survive in a most unpredictable world. Patsy remembers this grandmother as a very small woman, no taller than five feet and taking size four shoes. She wonders now if she were malnourished. She knows little of Olga's early life before she was sent to New York, but believes she was one of a large and impoverished family. It is possible that she was put out to adoption because she was not a boy. During her adolescence she fell in love with a boy, James, a year or two younger than herself. His family was in a business but, being a younger son, he would not inherit the firm so he decided to join the gold rush to Alaska to prospect. His quest for gold did not succeed and he settled down in an Alaskan town to edit the local newspaper. Olga and James were engaged before he went west to seek a fortune. She had the feeling that, although her betrothed was not a strong man, she would be able to make him succeed in whatever he did. Eventually she followed him to Alaska by train, sewing her trousseau on the journey.

Amanda was the eldest of Olga's three children and she then had a son and another daughter. They lived in a small town which clung to the edge of the wilderness. Patsy knows from photographs that her grandmother made enormous efforts to turn it into a respectable home, with

antimacassars on the backs of chairs, hand-sewn quilts for the
beds, shawls draped over the furniture, and a grand piano.
Her husband did not succeed as Olga had hoped, and she
then poured all her aspirations into her son and his future.
Patsy says he seems to have had unconditional love. Amanda
grew up knowing that she had the choice of becoming a
teacher or a librarian; there were no other options open to
her. Patsy commented that her grandmother was a judg-
mental woman and she thought that the same trait had come
out in her mother, Amanda. I began to understand the out-
pouring of personal talents into those around as a trait of the
grandmother as much as of the mother. That was the right
and only way for a woman to improve her own lot in life if
she were intelligent, strong and resourceful. During the First
World War, the family moved back to New York and later
they moved to California. Olga was in her mid-fifties when
her husband died. She had always been a competent seam-
stress, and for the first years after her husband's death she
continued to live alone in their bungalow and sew her own
clothes. Her beloved son's first marriage broke down and he
went to live with his mother. He was a keen fly fisherman
and his mother spent her time looking after him, doing the
cooking and making his special flies. But, in 1950, when his
mother was about seventy years old, he remarried. Olga
detested her new daughter-in-law. At the same time she lost,
not only her son, but also the job of looking after him which
provided her value. She gave up her home and spent the
next few years living half of each year with her daughters,
but she did not get on well with either of them. In 1954 her
three children joined together and rented a small property
for her, but she did not manage for long because she was
dementing. Patsy remembers her as a very rigid woman who

had to keep control of everybody and everything around her. She has a vivid memory of the large watch her grand-mother kept on a cord around her neck, which lay centrally over her waist. In her last years Olga started to wander and was constantly waiting for her husband to come home for his next meal.

Amanda was an outstandingly clever girl and finished her schooling in New York after her family's move there. In 1920 she was taken by her father to start at Berkeley University in California. The choice of that university antic-ipated the family's next move to San Diego in Southern California. For unknown reasons, her father arrived with her at university six weeks late, well into the first semester. Amanda then failed all her examinations and blamed her father for the things that went wrong; but she did not com-plain to him aloud either at that time or later. It seems to have remained as a festering grudge.

Amanda spent the next four years at Berkeley, and the rest of her life was defined by her intellectual ability and the culture she acquired during those years. She became en-meshed in the thoughts of the Bloomsbury Group, idealised the world of the English country cottage and wanted a few Japanese touches. She excelled in English literature and had a great interest in Shakespeare. After university she became a high-school teacher and must have excelled in this work because, many years later, after her death, her former pupils established a scholarship in her memory.

Amanda married a man who, in Patsy's words, needed to be held together and who subsequently betrayed her. Her husband, who had a problem with alcohol, had been mar-ried before and had a daughter by that marriage. She was thirty-two when she married and her husband thirty-eight.

Patsy describes him as dapper and charming; he always wore snazzy suits. Patsy was born two years after the marriage, but by the time of the birth the marriage had broken down and her father left his wife. Patsy heard that her mother had found her husband in bed with another woman while she was pregnant. She viewed her husband, Patsy's father, as a bastard that she must get rid of, and she never relinquished any of her passionate anger with him. When, years later, Patsy told her that he had died and she was going to his funeral, Amanda made no comment.

Amanda chose to be divorced from her husband when Patsy was still a baby. After the divorce the small child was put in the care of an English girl and Amanda went back to work. Amanda told Patsy that it was unusual for a mother to choose to be divorced and live with her daughter as a single parent. She made it clear to her daughter that the divorce was essential because her ex-husband was a drunken philanderer and a contemptible person. Amanda set out to be a perfect parent and show perfect love to her only child. She was not strict in the accepted sense of that word but she could control her daughter by raising an eyebrow. Patsy grew up with a strong sense of the need to please her mother and all those around her in order to be accepted.

Amanda created a remarkable world for her daughter's upbringing. It was a fantasy of her own invention, a re-creation of rural England in Southern California. Patsy describes the setting in which she grew up as a 'one woman Bloomsbury Group, enjoying the countryside and English culture and literature'. She was so successful in her creation that she made Patsy an object of envy to all her friends. But she made the friends very welcome and enjoyed being Patsy's hostess for any social gathering. She made a world of exciting ideas that stimulated all those around her. There was frequently a log fire burning in the traditionally English fireplace and mulled cider for Patsy's guests. Patsy and her friends were delighted to be treated as adults by this kind, intelligent and wise woman. Amanda would always intercede on behalf of other children with their parents, when she thought that the parents were being unreasonable. She provided four expensive ballgowns for her daughter, although money was tight, and her daughter could always be the best dressed girl at any gathering. She took her to football matches or any other event for which Patsy expressed a desire. But Patsy began to wonder if her mother was doing it for her own or her daughter's benefit, and if there were not a hidden demand to repay her mother for all the lavish generosity.

Amanda was able to make her small daughter feel responsible for the well-being of her only parent. On one occasion, when Patsy was about six years old, Amanda gave her twenty dollars to buy a bond when she went to school. This represented a lot of money and a big responsibility. The money was lost, but the child was unable to tell her mother because she felt that she had betrayed her. Amanda appeared to need her daughter as an equal, and to that end she structured and organised her own and her daughter's lives. The daughter became her reason for living, her pet and her companion. Patsy grew up realising that she was her mother's most valuable possession and main interest apart from her teaching.

However, Amanda knew that she herself was a local aristocrat because of the university from which she had graduated and her own intellectual superiority, and her daughter felt that she was being put into a most privileged position. There was music in Amanda's home, mainly Bartok and

Mahler, and Patsy comments that she had never heard Mozart until she was an adult. Amanda set the standards for herself and for those around her; they knew that if they fell from grace the situation was irredeemable. Certainly that is how Patsy saw it and still sees it. The world and life that Amanda wanted for herself and her daughter were set in the 1920s in England, and she did not want it to change. She had the charisma and the power to fake this world of her own creation. Amanda, and her mother before her, never seemed to be troubled by any doubts.

Amanda did not encourage Patsy to make contact with her father but, late in her childhood, she did spend part of each week with him during the school holidays. Although she enjoyed her father's company, and also that of his next three wives, she knew that she must not get too close to him because it threatened her mother.

Amanda made the largest investments of herself and her talents in four young people, two boys and two girls. She tried to model Patsy, but was unable to make her into the person she wanted, and Patsy still feels that her mother was immensely disappointed though this was never expressed by Amanda. Her other 'daughter', was physically the opposite of her biological one, fair, ethereal and artistic where her own daughter was dark, athletic and large framed. Amanda was more successful in forming her. This second daughter had an artistic career and remains immensely grateful to Amanda for the encouragement she gave. Of the two boys, one became a charming rogue and dropped out of conventional education; Amanda could accept this and even indulge it. The other, over whom she had a great influence, became a Roman Catholic convert and a priest. She found this very difficult to accept. She must have known that she had lost him irretrievably. He also remains profoundly grateful to her for her inspired teaching.

Patsy also excelled at school. Like her mother, she loved English literature but Amanda influenced her to major in a scientific subject at university. Amanda must have felt at this point that she was losing her control over her daughter. Patsy commented that her mother had better marbles than most people, but she also had the arrogance of somebody who knew herself to be intellectually superior. Beneath the certainty was contempt for underdogs and that included Jews, blacks, Mexicans and anybody whom she considered to be of inferior birth or intelligence. She hated organised religion and also, at various times, had battles with members of the medical profession. Both of these professional bodies appeared to threaten her power and desire to be in unopposed control. Patsy remembers an incident when she was three years old and had scarlet fever. The doctor did not agree with Amanda's assessment of the seriousness of the situation and Patsy can still remember her mother shaking with rage. She commented that her mother always felt that she was rejected by institutionalised power.

At university, Patsy changed courses many times and then announced her engagement to a man, without great wealth, from Scotland. Amanda was very angry and tried to impress on her daughter the sort of poverty that living in that city in Scotland would mean. When Patsy broke off the engagement and started going out with a wealthy Jew, her mother collaborated in the affair and bragged to her friends about her daughter's wealthy boyfriend. Patsy commented that her mother cannot have been pleased that she was marrying a Jew, but his wealth must have been a mitigating factor. Patsy married and had two children. Her mother adored the grandson, who could do no wrong, but disliked the grand-daughter intensely and mocked her.

The marriage failed and Patsy moved many hundreds of miles away. She saw her mother seldom and was much pre-occupied with remaking her own life. Patsy discovered that she was able to stand up to her mother and say ' No'. She thinks that this moment could have been the start of a new and different sort of relationship with her mother. Amanda retired within a year of the marriage breakdown and from that time, apart from one long holiday with a room-mate from her college days, she remained in the house where Patsy had been born and brought up. During those years the circle of highly intelligent people, who had taught with her at the community college, either died or moved away. Amanda told her daughter that she was the only one left, but she did not apparently grieve or show any emotion.

Patsy saw very little of her mother during the next few years. By the time they were able to see more of each other, Amanda had swung from being the one who was always in charge to being the one who was dependent. She cast her daughter in the role of the powerful and controlling mother. She would telephone her daughter many times during the day and night to ask her what she should do about every detail of her life. There did not seem to be any possibility of a relationship between equal and mature adults. Amanda spent most of the last year of her life in her daughter's home and the last months in a retirement home with nursing care.

Amanda died in 1987, but one of Patsy's friends told her that her mother's driving had scared her badly ten years earlier. She had apparently always been an erratic driver, but during the last years that she managed to live on her own and still drove, Patsy noticed unexplained green streaks along the side of Amanda's red car. When she asked her mother about these colours her mother said that something funny had happened to her vision. She kept seeing green cloudy stuff along the road so she just drove straight through it.

At one level it is easy to explain the bad driving and the later confusion by failing memory and concentration; but at another level the car represents, to some extent, the outer packaging of the person. A young man with his sports car, frequently a red one, identifies himself with the power and control of the car he drives. Did Amanda, still in charge of her car, but losing control over parts of herself and of those around her, try to implant her failing power on the boundaries of the road along which she was driving? I doubt if she could have driven more carefully, or voluntarily relinquished her car, any more than she could have given up her control over those around her. Caution, and a more balanced way, were not part of the pattern of her life.

I think of the legend of Icarus. In Greek mythology he was the son of the craftsman Daedalus, and he and his father were imprisoned on the island of Crete. In order to escape, Daedalus constructed a pair of wings for himself and a set for his son, which were attached to the shoulders by wax. They started off, and Daedalus instructed his son that he must fly neither too high nor too low; but Icarus was disobedient and flew too near the sun and the wax melted. His wings dropped off and he fell into the sea and was drowned. Amanda did not know a balanced way, of success and failure, loss as well as gain. She was an expert in making her own creation and controlling it.

The first time that I visited California I was amazed at the way in which man had established his control over every detail of himself and of his environment. I had the impression that anything could be made or altered, given sufficient money, power and skill. That included changing the entire appearance of a street or the shape of a body. But man does not have control over death. Amanda was a high-flyer who invented her own world. I wondered if she had also taken on the moral tenets of the Bloomsbury Group and chosen to defy conventional morality. She was not fearful of shocking people. The two things of supreme importance to her were bringing up her daughter as her chosen companion, and her teaching. In the world which she created, she had great power, and could inspire other people to do the things which she most wanted for them, and in as far as it was what they most desired for themselves, they remember her with respect and affection. But, unlike a member of the original Blooomsbury Group, she did not write creatively or paint. Anybody in a position of authority, a doctor, or a minister of religion, or even an adult man living with her as an equal adult, would have threatened her control and authority, and she allowed no such person to remain near her.

I thought again of my image of a crowded stage and the blank space where the principal character, Amanda, should have been. After many hours of listening to Patsy's narrative, and more hours of thinking and writing, that blank remains, although I have discovered much of her in the young people nearest to her. For Amanda it was always seed-time, a time for the scattering of her ideas and a dispersal of herself and her talents. There never seemed to be a right time for gathering in and harvest before death.

I am left with a strong sense of her isolation. This was reinforced when I heard some extracts from tapes on an answerphone from the last year of Amanda's life, while she was staying in her daughter's house. The theme running through them is that nobody is at home. Amanda is trying to take messages for Patsy who is not at home. She has no idea where she has gone or when she will be back and does not know how to get in touch with her. There is a sense of speaking into a blank space, where there is nobody present, and she does not expect an answer, and has no hope of a relationship. The voice that talks to her at the other end of the telephone is not expecting her and does not know her. Sometimes the person on the phone does know her and attempts to make contact, but Amanda does not remember the voice or to whom it belongs. Overall, there is a chilling sense of strangers making sounds but nothing having any meaning. There are bits of information but it does not fit together. There are arrangements for a meeting at an airport which nobody knows. Where is the terminal? Don't know. Which terminal do we meet at? I don't know. I don't know the airport. There are scattered news items that do not fit together. Listen, listen. Can you hear me? Are you there? A voice crying in a lost place. No love, no affection, no relationship.

Can I imagine what it is like to dement and lose control of the world that, for all my life, I have, through my own intellect and hard work, been able to control? It could be like a tangle of wires and flexes that cannot be fitted together in the right way to make the power go on flowing through them. At one level, one can say this is exactly what happens when the neurotransmitters, like acetylcholine, are deficient and can no longer relay the messages. But in another way, and at another level, it could be like a nightmare from which there can be no waking and release.

In outer reality I have a deadline for the completion of a

book and I am trying to come to terms with a new word-processor. I wake sweating at three in the morning because the computer is smoking and the screen has gone blank. I can no longer impress what I want through the keyboard into the world of the computer. Suddenly the screen is in revolt and it starts talking to me. But then I wake up. This is the world of nightmare, and most of us can remember dreams or nightmares of a similar sort. But if one could not wake up and look at the entanglement and compare it with the outer reality, but had to go on blindly caught up in the inner reality, the dream, I believe, would feel like dementia, disintegration.

Amanda had been damaged, devalued and isolated very early in her life, and had survived by dint of her own intelligence, hard work and ability to create her own life. She acquired the power to create her own world in which she could operate with some degree of safety; but in the doing and achieving she could never relinquish any power or show any weakness. She never showed sadness or expressed feeling about her losses. Perhaps she did not dare to expose the part of herself that might not be in control. With such everlasting and superhuman effort there could eventually be a burn-up in her own inner centre.

Through Amanda's family there runs a strain of missing parents and weak fathers. Her mother lost both her parents at the age of three and had to survive with substitute ones in a strange country, speaking a different language. She grew up to be a dominant woman who married a weak husband. Amanda despised her own father and blamed him for the things that had gone wrong in her early life. She then seems to have set the stage of her life for a solo performance. She married a man who was a frail person and never played any important role in her life after he had fathered her daughter. From then on he was banned and exiled. Did she need to acquire so much power in order to survive her childhood? Did the same power remain unchallenged because there was no strong, wise man in her life? Could she have listened to a man's voice?

I wonder if Amanda was the 'too good' mother, who gave endlessly of herself and invested her talents in other people. I have a feeling that those around Amanda feel in her debt. Eventually everything was in some way tied up outside herself and there was nothing left to gather in for her personal harvest. She was then lost, blank and emptied out into a state of meaninglessness.

Chapter 5

Alice

I listened to two accounts of Alice's life, one from her niece, Jane, and the other from her sister-in-law, Theresa. During the first session, Jane was alone and the only narrator; during the second session both Jane and Theresa were present but, for most of the time, Theresa was the narrator. It was interesting for me to hear this narrative from two viewpoints and two generations; both women saw parts of Alice's life which had previously been hidden from them. The meetings were on two successive days in a friend's house in the mid-west of the USA. I had met neither of the women before the first session and initially I was apprehensive about having two narrators in one session.

Neither of the narrators was genetically related to Alice and, from the start of the narrations, I was aware of a greater degree of objectivity than in the previous narration about Amanda; but there was less objectivity in Jane's account because, I believe, of her role as surrogate daughter. Awareness of these differences triggered more thoughts about objectivity and involvement, and the reasons for a familial pattern of Alzheimer's disease that was not necessarily genetic.

Jane told me that her aunt and uncle should have had children because they would have been such marvellous parents. It was clear, from early in the meeting, that Jane had been, for them, a surrogate daughter. Alice and her husband,

Ted, had no living offspring. She had four pregnancies, of which only one went the full time, and the baby died at three days old. She also had at least two miscarriages. The family and their spouses were and are practising Roman Catholics. Ted was the eldest of four brothers. One brother, Jane's father, had six children, another brother had seven and the fourth died early in life. Jane felt that, for Alice, child-lessness must have been heartbreaking, but she was never aware of any sadness. As a child, Jane loved visiting her aunt and uncle and with them she always felt herself wrapped in love. She described Ted as a clever man who also excelled in sport. He enjoyed the company of children and was end-lessly active. When he was not being physically active he would sit and talk. It was clear that Jane enjoyed this very special relationship with her aunt and uncle, which must have been different from being one of six children in her own home.

Alice was born in 1911 and brought up in a busy mid-west town in the USA. She was an only child, brought up mainly by her mother because her father was frequently away on business trips. Her Roman Catholicism was, Jane believed, always important for her; and even if she was ill and, later, when she was dementing, she still wanted to get to mass. Jane's view of Alice was an idealised one of a woman who was beautiful, clever, loving and full of brilliant conversation. She had trained as a schoolteacher and Jane said that she could talk about anything at all. She had loved teaching but gave it up when she got married. Jane described Ted as always a bit on the 'wild side'. Alice was less physi-cally active and Jane remembers her hands, because she always wore a lot of jewellery and many rings. Her nails were painted and she smoked. The elegant hands, the many rings, the rattling bracelets and the cigarettes made an impression on Jane as a child; and she remembers that Alice was always well dressed. She saw nothing negative in her at all. It looked like a picture of a perfect mother–daughter relationship, with no dark side at all. Jane faithfully filled the role of a loving, uncritical and dutiful daughter for the whole of Alice's life.

Jane's mother was ill when she was a small child and she and one of her brothers were sent to Alice and Ted. At this time she remembers Ted as the one who was responsible for them, coming to see what they were doing in the garden. Alice allowed him to be in charge of them.

Jane thinks that Ted may have minded more about not having children than Alice, but he never spoke about it. Through his church he became interested in the boy scouts and coached them in sport. Jane thought that he was very happy when his son, Peter, was born but three days later the baby had died. Jane felt that it was a close marriage but she did not think that they spoke together about their losses and sadness. Jane thought of Ted as more sensitive than Alice and knew that he would do and say nothing to hurt her feelings. Ted and his brother, Michael, who later married Theresa, had a warm and close relationship, but Jane's father had always been different and more remote. Jane enjoyed the closeness and warmth with Alice and Ted, and had a sense of family with them that she did not have with her own.

Jane left school and started training as a nurse at a hospital near to her aunt and uncle. She saw a lot of them during these years. She married and moved away but later returned, and over the next years had five children. Ted and Alice were in a special position as great-uncle and great-aunt and also godparents to her children. They attended confirmations, first communions and school functions. Jane's position as surrogate daughter became more established. When Alice was dementing and unable to stay in her own home, even with Ted's unfailing help, Jane made space in her home for them to move in. They stayed there until Alice died and then, six months later, Ted died.

During the second session, when Theresa was the principal narrator, we saw a very different view of Alice. I say 'we' because I believe there were as many surprises for Jane as for myself. Theresa and Michael, Ted's younger brother, were already engaged when Ted brought Alice to meet them. Theresa, who seemed an intuitive woman, had an instant impression that Alice was a cold and unfeeling person. After Ted and Alice were married, they lived with her parents for a year while Alice supervised the building of their home. She gave up teaching after the marriage and stayed at home; Theresa thought that she had her own money. The house was described by both Jane and Theresa as very beautiful, like a Hansel and Gretel house, with an enormous fireplace. Theresa and Michael would go to see them after an evening out, when they would all sit and talk in front of the big fire. Theresa became more accepting of her sister-in-law, but describes her as a 'feisty' woman who was never afraid to state her opinion and would always call a spade a spade. She was an only child, of Irish origin and full of good humour. Theresa thought that she did know about sadness but she never showed it and always behaved in a very upbeat way. A year after Ted and Alice moved into their new home, Theresa and Michael got married and came to live near them. A year later Theresa had her first child, and two years later a second; and it was clear that Alice and Ted enjoyed seeing the babies. Then Alice had her first pregnancy, but there was something wrong with her kidneys and she lost the baby. Theresa does not know if, or how much, she was saddened by the loss; Alice never spoke about it or showed her grief. She had three more pregnancies but buried all the babies. Ted always seemed to be with one or other of Theresa's children which was useful because Michael was not an active, sporty sort of person.

When Theresa was pregnant with her fifth child, the last but one, she accepted a teaching position in a Roman Catholic school. After she had the baby she wanted to stay at home for a year, and asked Alice if she would like to take the job over. Alice accepted it and was pleased to be back at work after so many years at home. She was a university graduate and enjoyed the work, but after five years the school had difficulty in paying all the staff and Alice decided that she would leave and teach in a public-sector school. She remained there, teaching fifth-grade pupils, until she retired about twenty years later. She was described as a brilliant teacher. She was always greeted by her present and past pupils when she was around the town, during the years that she was working in the school and for the rest of her active life. All her pupils were happy to claim and recognise her and declare that she was the best teacher that they had had. Theresa thinks this was partly because she was always very smartly dressed. Neither Jane nor Theresa was certain, but it was possible that Alice had to retire before the normal age because her memory was failing.

Shortly before Alice retired, Theresa and Michael and all their children moved several thousand miles away to California. Theresa knows that this affected Alice and Ted very much. Theresa said that her children always seemed to belong as much to Alice as to herself. Alice and Ted did once go to stay in California, but otherwise they met two or three times a year when Theresa and her family came back to their original home in the mid-west, which they kept.

In retirement, Alice and Ted got involved with sport of various sorts. Ted played golf, they both played bowls and went to football matches. Then Jane and her family moved near again and her family filled the void which the departure of Theresa's family had left.

After her last disastrous pregnancy, and the baby that lived for only three days, Alice was told that she had high blood pressure and should have no more pregnancies. She spoke with Theresa about adopting a baby; but she decided not to, and Theresa thinks she made that decision because of her hypertension. Theresa said that, apart from the conversation about adoption, Alice had never at any time spoken about the lost babies or shown any sadness. Theresa is obviously an open and receptive person who would have kept her confidence but, although she made herself available, Alice did not speak and there would have been nobody else to whom she could have spoken. It must have been difficult for Alice to have had a sister-in-law with six children while she herself was childless, but Theresa thinks it may have been of some comfort to her that she had been to a more academic university and had a better degree than Theresa had. She seems to have been happier after she resigned herself to being childless and started teaching. She secretly helped poor children with white dresses for their confirmations.

Theresa described Alice as a reserved person who never wept. Ted was the only person to whom she had ever been close. She did not seem to have had friends of her own. Their friends had always been his friends whom she accepted and welcomed into her home. Theresa said that Jane's mother did not like Alice because she felt that she could never get close to her. When she and Jane's father went to the town where Alice and Ted lived, they would always avoid having to stay with them.

Jane had not known anything about Alice's father until this meeting. She was surprised when she discovered that Theresa remembered him well. She said that he had always been a difficult man, an adventurer, involved in inventions and pioneer work. I asked if anybody else in the family had developed Alzheimer's disease. Theresa replied that Alice's father had been put in an asylum when he was about sixty years old. It was said that one night he had attacked Ted with a knife. Jane had never heard about this. There must have been a sense of deep shame and secrecy about this in the family. Obviously both Ted and Alice knew, but although Jane had, for many years, been closer to Alice than anybody else, she had known nothing of it until now. Theresa said that Alice's father had always been uncommunicative and solitary. It seems possible that he did dement; he does not seem to have had a previous history of mental illness, and he did not recover and return home. Alice's relationship with her father, and the trauma of his mental illness, were shut away and denied in the same way as her sorrow over the dead babies. I had the feeling that Alice kept everything in her life in separate compartments.

At around the time of Alice's retirement she started making many errors in paying accounts and was muddled when writing cheques. Up until then she had managed their money, but at this point Ted took over. Jane was surprised when she visited them to find Ted doing the cooking, but he explained that, if he left it for Alice, everything was burnt. Earlier in the marriage, Alice's mother had lived with them and at that time she always did the cooking. In some ways Alice was prepared to be the child and be looked after.

In the final years of Alice's life, she and Ted went to live in Jane's home because, as she explained, she and her husband had a large home, her family had left and, in a way, Ted and Alice became her family. Earlier in life she was their surrogate daughter, emotionally dependent on them; later in life the pattern was reversed and Ted and Alice were dependent on her. During the first year they shared the home, Ted and Alice ate in their own part of the house but later they all ate together because it was easier for Ted. For part of the time, Alice went to a day centre and Ted was still able to play golf; Jane took and fetched her on her way to and from her own part-time teaching job.

Until Alice demented, she was the one who was always in control, but afterwards she became totally dependent on Ted. She would not allow Theresa to bath her. She wanted nobody to do anything involving close bodily contact, apart from Ted. To him she became like a baby. Theresa commented that it seemed a strong bond of mutual dependency; in the end he cared for her like his own child. It seemed that increasingly Alice and Ted became interdependent and had a relationship with each other that did not include anybody else. Until her death, Alice always recognised Ted. If he went out and somebody else was looking after her she would ask repeatedly 'Where's Ted?' Late in her life, when she could make no movement without help, Ted would help her to the bathroom, dress her and feed her. She always had to kiss the top of Ted's head before she could be helped to do anything. Jane said so much of Alice had gone, but Ted always responded to her as though she were still there. After her death he became very depressed and died six months later. It was as though their lives were so interdependent that he could not live without her.

The empty space

Despite two different viewpoints on the life of Alice, I realised that I still knew remarkably little about her. Like Amanda, she remained largely a blank patch. Jane's account of Alice told me more about Jane's own warmth and positive outlook on life, than about Alice. Here I saw the lack of objectivity in a description from somebody who only saw the light, and never the dark, side of a person. Theresa's account was objective and gave a very different view of this woman and her restricted life. From these two glimpses of Alice, I began to imagine what her life was like and what it felt like to be Alice. This view depends, to a large extent, on my own imagination.

She was an only daughter; nobody knows if that was from parental choice. Her father was frequently absent and was described as a difficult man. I wonder if, very early in life, she made herself a small isolated place from which she could look out on life without relating to it too closely. She would then be able to distance herself from her feelings; strong feelings, and particularly sad ones, need a secure environment to become accepted. There is much evidence that Alice had a great capacity for avoiding or denying all strong feeling. She did not express her sadness over the loss of her babies, and it is likely that even Ted was kept at a distance from her sorrow. Eventually they were totally dependent on each other, but that was only after the onset of her disintegration.

While thinking and writing about her, I am aware of her

beautiful house, with its log fire in the enormous fireplace, her elegant appearance and in particular her bejewelled hands; but I am left with a gap about the essential person who was Alice. Theresa described her as an upbeat lady. She married into a large, warm and child-loving family, and was nourished by Ted and by the two women with whom I had spoken. She was talented at providing a home where she welcomed other people's children, but never became totally committed to her own family, or to the mourning of her own family.

I have found myself using the word 'surrogate' many times while I write the account of Alice. In the *Shorter Oxford English Dictionary*, 'surrogate' has a number of different meanings including 'a person or thing that acts for or takes the place of another; a substitute'. Was Alice, an only child with an absent father, a substitute for a whole family of children and also possibly a substitute for the missing husband? I saw a similar picture in Amanda's life and the way in which she brought up her daughter. I wonder if the small child, who is cast as a substitute very early in life, is never able to take over as principal character in her own life to live her own individual story.

Could Alice have been alienated from her own self, her own and entirely personal inner space, very early in her life? She developed a great ability to fill in for those around her, whether it was as mother or teacher. In the inner empty space of somebody who dements, could there be something set in stone, cold, hard and unyielding, instead of somewhere warm, receiving and secure, with the capability for joy and sorrow? Is it because there was no stable home and the infant was never valued in its own right? Possibly an early 'chill' factor in the centre could make the person more likely to disintegrate? If that was the picture in very early life, this person would be vulnerable. I do not believe, however, that this is a final and irrevocable state, because I think there are choices along the way, which I see in all the stories.

Chapter 6

Elspeth

Elspeth was born in Glasgow in 1908. Her mother was a Yorkshire woman who had been orphaned at the age of eighteen and was then taken in by Scottish friends. Her father was a stonemason from Angus. Elspeth's son, Rob, remembered that he loved literature and poetry and had many relatives who were interesting characters. Rob's grandmother died young, at about the age of fifty, from bronchial trouble. He thinks that she had brothers and sisters but was separated from them after her parents' death. Rob remembers her as an isolated and beautiful character. Elspeth was the middle child of three though the eldest, a boy, had died of diphtheria before she was born. At the age of three, Elspeth had scarlet fever and was in an isolation hospital for three months. When she spoke about this to Rob, she described herself as inconsolable. She said that from that time, and for the rest of her life, she always felt cold. There was another girl, four years younger than Elspeth, who was a very different character. Rob describes his mother as always upright, orderly and well dressed; but he described the younger sister as a harum-scarum.

One of Elspeth's fondest memories of her childhood was of long walks with her father. He always had a book of poetry in one pocket and a bar of chocolate in the other. Rob remembers his grandfather as an eccentric man who was large and white bearded; late in his life he kept his open fire burning with a very long tree-trunk. As the end burned in the fire, he pushed the trunk further in. He was always up early, active and energetic, and died at the age of seventy, after eight days' illness. His mind did not disintegrate and he seems to have been mentally active all his life.

The dead son was talked about a great deal both when Elspeth was a child and, later, when Rob was a child. He seems to have been an angelic presence who, in his invisible way, had a profound influence on the family members who survived him. His memory remained vividly alive. There were many pictures of the dead child, and Elspeth felt that her father never recovered from that loss. She felt that she had taken the dead child's place as she grew up and she saw this substitution, surrogacy, as a privileged role. She knew that she provided some security for her parents, but she never had any sense that they agonised over their son's death or were overprotective of her. It was more likely that, being an uptight family, any strong feelings were kept very much under control.

Elspeth was very clever and did well at school, but at that time it was considered that daughters did not need a lot of education After she left school she did a secretarial course and passed her examinations with flying colours. Her son never heard her speak about the things she could have done with more training, and she was not the sort of person to have regrets about what might have been. She was employed by a large industrial manufacturer and did so well that she was offered promotion and a job in London when she was eighteen. That was in 1926, and her parents would not allow her to take the position because they thought that it would be bad for her. She remained in the same firm, and a few years later was asked out by a man who was in a more junior position. He was shorter than she was and also three years younger. She was so embarrassed by this discrepancy in their ages that she kept it secret even from her son; he only discovered it accidentally when he was in his twenties. They were married in 1938, when she was thirty and he was twenty-seven. Rob's father saw her mother as an exalted person and he felt very daring in asking her out. Elspeth was attractive and had many boyfriends, but her mind seems to have been principally on her work. Rob added that she remained an attractive and smart woman until her dying day. Her husband stayed in the firm after the marriage, but Elspeth had to leave because it was not acceptable that a married woman should continue in employment. After the war started in 1939 she was able to go back to work, and remained there until the end of the war. Rob thinks there was some sadness that they did not have children during those first years of the marriage, but life was tough and they spent many nights in air-raid shelters.

Their first, and only, child, Rob, was born in 1946, a year after the war ended. It was a difficult birth and Elspeth had a Caesarean section. Following the operation she remained unconscious for a number of days. Her husband was told not to celebrate because neither his wife nor son might live. There were many complications, but both she and the baby survived though she did not see her baby for a fortnight. She was not able to breastfeed and she was told that she must never have another baby. Elspeth and the baby remained in hospital for many weeks and the father was excluded. From that time, the relationship between the mother and baby became stronger than a normal mother-child bonding, with the father remaining a peripheral figure. Elspeth became the central figure in the family and had a great influence over her son.

Rob's father was an extrovert and made friends easily. He would call people by their Christian names at the first meeting, which was not the normal custom amongst the people he and his wife met during that time in Scotland. Rob knew, at a very early age, that he must find his own way of living in order to have any existence separate from his mother. He became uncommunicative to his mother, entered into his own world, invented his own games and companions, and preferred to play alone in his own room. He had no relationship with his father. Rob was aware, from early on, of the stresses within the family relationships. Although he wanted to be independent of his mother, he knew that he had a more important place in her affections than his father. His mother's need of him forced him into the ambivalent position of both wanting to be a good and affectionate son, with an exclusive relationship with his mother, and at the same time keep her at arm's length.

When Rob was three years old, Elspeth's father came to live with them and she looked after him until his death two years later. Rob remembers his grandfather with affection. He thinks that those two years must have been full of work, but also of warmth, for Elspeth.

Rob started at primary school about the time of his grandfather's death, while the family was still living in Glasgow, but when he was eight years old the family moved to Dundee because his father, still with the same firm, was offered and accepted promotion. Rob was excited about the move, though apprehensive about changing his school where he was thriving, happy and successful. Rob remembers that Elspeth did not survive that move at all well. It was the first time that she had lived away from Glasgow, and she became agitated and depressed.

During the years in Glasgow, Elspeth went to the Presbyterian church and took Rob, but his father never went. She stopped attending church after the move to Dundee but Rob requested that he be allowed to attend Sunday school. Rob thinks that after the move Elspeth's life was empty. Her husband worked hard in a more demanding job, her son was at school and she did not have a job of her own. She did not enjoy cooking or home-making, although she liked her clothes and her home to be elegant. She spent a little time with her neighbours and Rob remembers that his parents did sometimes have friends in their home. But on the whole, the early years in Dundee must have been empty and lonely for Elspeth. Then, when Rob was in his early teens, Elspeth was asked to run her husband's office, and suddenly she came back into her own world again and thrived. There were, of necessity, big changes at home, and she worried that she was never at home when her son got back from school; but he went to neighbours until she got home and he also thrived. Elspeth ran the office and did the firm's accounts brilliantly well and won much praise for her organisation.

During the holidays Rob also went to the neighbours and sometimes he went into town to the office. Elspeth continued to be concerned about what she saw as neglect of her son and was unaware that he enjoyed this change in his family's circumstances. She retired from work when she was fifty-five and Rob was eighteen. By this time her husband was the senior person in the Dundee office, in charge of a staff of twenty. They were well off financially, and moved to an exclusive residential area of Dundee. There was a certain amount of business entertaining and Elspeth enjoyed occasions at elegant restaurants. Rob's father did some travelling in Scotland and England and occasionally he took Rob with him, which Rob enjoyed. Every year the family had a holiday in Switzerland in the same comfortable hotel. Rob thinks that, although both of his parents earned good salaries, they probably lived up to the limit of their income. Rob went away to college when he was twenty-one, having lived at home until then. Three years later his father went into hospital with a severe cough and was diagnosed as having lung cancer. He remained in hospital for some time and Elspeth became depressed. Her husband came out of hospital and had six months remission from his disease. He managed to help Rob move into his first flat. A few months later, he died aged fifty-nine; Elspeth at that time was sixty-two. At the funeral there was an enormous number of people. Rob was surprised because he had not realised how many friends his father had or how popular he had been. He also wondered how his mother would survive. She became acutely depressed and wanted to take her life.

Elspeth was rescued, for the second time, from an unbearable gap in her life by a job offer. On this occasion the job was as secretary to a social work organisation. She was capable of doing the work and thoroughly enjoyed her new responsibilities. She organised her department so well that, when her boss moved away, she was left in charge. She took over the day-to-day running of the organisation, and also the design of the training courses. It was an ideal occupation for her and her son rejoiced that once again his mother's abilities were suitably harnessed. She went on with this work until she was seventy, when she was forced to retire.

After her retirement she helped with a number of charities, often as treasurer. By this time she was again actively involved with the Presbyterian church, although at times she wanted to go to the Episcopalian church to which her son belonged, but in some way she would not allow herself to go. Her father had been an Episcopalian but had stopped going to church before Elspeth's birth. Perhaps this was connected with the death of his son. One of Elspeth's uncles had been an Episcopalian priest and Rob feels that his own love of Anglo-Catholicism was 'in the blood', but his mother resisted the pull and could not, or would not, allow herself to go to the Episcopal church. Rob had been frightened of telling her of his own leanings during his adolescence. He had a great talent for music and, as an organist, he became closely involved with high-church worship. His mother could accept that he had left the Presbyterian church because of his music, and although she made no objection she did not express approval until she demented. When they were on holiday she would accompany her son to the Episcopalian church and he thought that the worship gave her pleasure.

After her second retirement, Elspeth continued with charity work and helped in an old people's home, but she was very lonely and found life empty. It must have been like another bereavement, a loss of the things she found important. At this time she started reading. She had one close woman friend, but the woman remarried and that was another loss. Elspeth was found to have something wrong with her heart and was put on beta blockers, but she had a bad reaction to them. She struggled on for two or three years before she saw a consultant privately and he gave her a pacemaker; after that she was physically well again. When she was seventy-four years old she moved from the family home in Dundee to a smaller flat.

Elspeth met a much younger woman through her charity work, and they both decided they would like to improve their bridge. She already played a little but now she became seriously interested and played many afternoons a week. She met many other bridge players but remained most friendly with the woman with whom she had started the serious commitment.

Rob said that he noticed that she became increasingly authoritarian. Always right-wing in politics, she now developed extreme views. Her son thought that, at the time of her eightieth birthday party, she was becoming a bitter and angry old lady.

The following year, when she was staying in her son's home, she came to his bedroom one night complaining that her room was haunted and that she had lost her alarm clock and her credit cards. Rob found her missing property in her room and reassured her. Looking back, he realises that by this time she was becoming confused and forgetful. She became increasingly stubborn and refused to accept advice or help. On one occasion, while staying with her son, she insisted on carrying a heavy tray laden with good china from the kitchen into the garden. She dropped it and all the china was smashed.

On her next birthday she was taken by Rob and a cousin to stay in a hotel. The morning of her birthday they took presents to her bedroom and found her very distressed because she said that her skirt was missing from her wardrobe. She had always been, and remained, very clothes conscious. Rob looked around her room and in the wardrobe but he could not find the missing skirt. Elspeth was so sure that it had been stolen that Rob felt compelled to report it to the hotel reception The owner of the hotel was sensitive and tactful and was able to have a thorough search done of Elspeth's room while she was at breakfast. The skirt was found in the wardrobe.

From that time she became increasingly confused. For example, she would telephone Rob, much concerned that a long dead friend had not telephoned her. She came to stay with Rob in his new home and got lost in the house, which was on several storeys. She got to the basement and could not find her way back again. She had never like television, but at this visit she insisted that it was turned off. Before that she would tolerate her son watching for a short time.

Rob was telephoned to say that his mother had fallen and was in hospital. She had gone shopping because, as she had explained to a friend, her son and her father were coming to lunch. On her return she had fallen down with the shopping on her front doorstep. The following night she fell out of bed and spent the night on the floor, having wetted herself. The doctor was called and she was admitted to a geriatric hospital. When her son arrived, she was hallucinating and told him that a friend had come but would not speak to her. She warned him to be careful what he said because other people were listening. She had difficulty remembering which bed was hers. The hospital staff tried to persuade her to go into a home where she could be properly cared for, but she was adamant that she was all right, and insisted on going back to her flat. She went home without any social services support and she started to telephone her son, day and night. She would tell him that she had cooked the food for him and his father but that his father had not come in for it. One night she telephoned to tell Rob that she was unable to understand why his father had not spoken to her. He had been in bed with her the previous night but he left without speaking to her.

After another night on the floor, and a fire from a

burned pan, her doctor arranged for her to be admitted to a home. During her time in the nursing home she became sweet natured, affectionate and always grateful for the care she was given. She was gracious to the care assistants and addressed them as 'nurse'. She acquired a *grande dame* persona which gave her a special position. Although the home was very expensive, many of the people there were local and not well educated. Elspeth continued to dress well and would ask a friend to go out and buy her new dresses. She employed somebody to come in and do her hair. She had no idea of the passing of time and no longer fretted about the non-appearance of her husband and son. She was allowed to go out on her own for walks, although she did sometimes have falls and frequently got lost. Rob went to see her as often as possible and took her to see her own flat. At those times she would ask when she would be able to go home, but she was content to leave again with her son and return to the nursing home. She always recognised her son and managed to write letters to him, but they were confused. The most painful moment for Rob was when it became necessary to sell her flat in order to pay for the nursing home, and he had to ask Elspeth to sign the forms for him to have the power of attorney. She was a woman who had been accustomed to handling not only her own affairs but those of offices. She had known about the minutiae of business contracts and she made him read out every word on the form, although it is unlikely that she understood. She was worried that if she signed the document somebody, her son, could then turn her out of her rightful home. She signed the form and then asked him to give her the cheque book because she needed to send for a new dress. It seems such a characteristic way for her to make it clear that, in spite of everything, she was still in charge of her own destiny.

After a year in the home, she spilt a teapot over her thighs and was badly burned. She was taken to the hospital burns unit and eventually had a skin graft. She continued to have a lot of pain from where the graft was taken. She did not understand what had happened and became increasingly confused. While she was recovering, a friend came and took her out for a walk. She insisted on wearing high-heeled shoes, and while she walked along the beach by the estuary she fell and broke her hip. The hip was repaired but she could not be coaxed to walk again. She got weaker and very thin and died in hospital.

Familiar themes

Elspeth grew up under the shadow of a dead brother, and she realised early in her life that she was a substitute for him. Although she saw this position as a privileged one, it must have made it more difficult for her to become herself. The role of a substitute, or surrogate, must have caused an alienation from her true self, because of the need to compensate her parents for not being the brother.

Elspeth was clever and that made her special, but she was not given the opportunity to study for a profession. She was not allowed to accept promotion in her firm and go away from her family to London. Rob said that she was not the sort of person to have thought or spoken about the 'might-have-beens', but she must have either felt or denied feelings of deprivation. She excelled when she was in a position where she could be responsible and organise; this was her salvation when she suffered a loss, for instance, after the move to Dundee, and after her retirement and the death of her husband.

She wanted elegance around her, particularly in her clothes, her hair and her home and she enjoyed the benefits that money brought her. It was her love of high-heeled shoes and her insistence on wearing them that contributed to the tragedy of her final fall and fractured hip. When her mind started to disintegrate she thought she had been robbed of a skirt and her credit card and these were representations of her most valued outer possessions.

Elspeth had the early experience of a missing, dead child, and it was a long time after marriage that she had her first baby. At that time, she nearly died, the baby was in danger, and she was told that she must have no more babies. Once again there is the shadow of a dead child. She never expressed her feelings, apart from her description of her three desolate months in a fever hospital at the age of three, and her stark statement that after that time she always felt cold. Was this coldness literal or was it a numbing of her feelings? Was this coldness perpetuated throughout her life? Her strongest feelings were for her son but her son had to keep her at arm's length for his own survival. The husband was always in second place to the son and I intuit that he was less intelligent than she was, in addition to being younger, shorter and, initially, in an inferior position in the firm.

Elspeth must have been brought up in an atmosphere of anxiety because she followed the brother who had died from diphtheria and then herself had scarlet fever, which was still very much a killer disease. She was the replacement for her brother, and the threat to her life must have been terrifying for her parents.

For Elspeth an empty space was a terrifying void. Her chosen option for filling the space was a job which was clearly a recognisable and valued entity. But time ran out for her in that role, and she was made to retire. She then continued her pattern of busy-ness with reading and bridge and voluntary work. For her, the empty space either had to be filled with organised activity or, if it were left open, she fell into it and was overtaken by depression. There is evidence that she preferred her space so full that there was no possible chink in it.

CHAPTER 7

Bob

Bob was the third and youngest child of elderly parents. His wife, Anne, describes his family as scrupulously honest and hard working, who always paid any debt without delay. He had a loving mother who was protective towards him, probably because he was the youngest. The early example of his parents lasted throughout his life; if he saw an unfamiliar pencil he wanted to know where it had come from. Bob's father was strict and did not show affection. Anne described him as a 'nothingness man' with high principles. His wife, Bob's mother, always tried to keep the peace and make everybody around her happy. Their house was small but she tried to give Bob and Anne space when they were courting, and was always ready to pack them up a picnic meal if they wanted to go out.

Bob and Anne first met when he was twenty-six and she was a few years younger. He had completed his apprenticeship as a bricklayer and worked for a large building firm. Anne had completed her training as an infant teacher. Their family homes were a few miles apart in a rural area of England, but they had not met as children. Bob was keen on photography and belonged to a club, enjoyed ballroom dancing and liked the solo occupation of fishing.

They married after a courtship of two years and lived in rented accommodation. They continued to work full-time in their own jobs. Bob decided to build their home himself and they managed to find a plot of a third of an acre on the outskirts of a nearby market town. Anne knew that Bob would never take risks, certainly not financial ones, and would not take any step until he could see the way forward clearly. He drew up the plans for their house; when they were passed, he built the brick shell, did the plumbing and had advice and some help with the electrical work. When he could not work outside on the building he worked in the cellar of their apartment, making window and door frames and, later, the kitchen table, four chairs, shelves, a coffee table and the cupboards. He never wanted to pay out more than they could earn, but eventually he did need a small mortgage. After two years of this round-the-clock labour they moved into their new home, although there were no floors and the kitchen had no fitments. Anne said that the hard work they shared gave them both much pleasure and they still had the time and energy to see their friends and, after the move, to have friends to stay. The large garden also needed their attention. It was part of a field and had to be cleared of thistles and spear grass before it was possible to make a garden.

Two years after the move their first child was born at home. The baby was weak and needed oxygen. Anne was told not to send out cards announcing the birth but to wait. Fortunately all went well, and the baby thrived. Soon after the birth, Bob's mother got ill and her mind became confused. Bob brought both his parents to live with his family because he thought it would be easier for Anne to cope. Bob was very fond of his mother and found it hard to see her ill and deteriorating. After her death, the family decided that Bob's father would never manage on his own, and they arranged for him to spend half the year with Bob and Anne and the other half with his daughter and her husband. Far from being authoritarian, at this stage of his life he became passive and easily accommodated. He died while with Bob and Anne, about six years after his wife.

Soon after his death, Anne's parents were no longer able to cope on their own and Bob and Anne helped them to find a bungalow nearby. Bob did an enormous amount of rebuilding on the bungalow and made a new bathroom and kitchen. Anne's mother lived there for six months and died of a stroke; her father died a year later.

Bob appears to have remained very busy and unemotional throughout this series of bereavements. Following the first birth, Anne had two miscarriages. However, she knew that she could not share her distress with her husband because he did not believe in depression. Eventually she did have another pregnancy that went the full time, and the baby was delivered at home. However, the baby, a boy, was very jaundiced and Anne's instinct told her that he also had something much more serious wrong with him. About a week after the birth, their doctor told Bob that the baby had a serious genetic abnormality and would not live. The doctor left Bob to tell Anne; in her heart she already knew. The baby died when he was sixteen days old. Bob seemed to 'blank out' and could not show his feelings, although Anne thinks now that he minded very much. Anne wanted to cry but knew that she must do it alone. She comments now that, in those days, nobody talked about bereavement or suggested counselling. She does not know whether it could have helped them to speak together about their grief; as it was, they remained isolated. She decided that it would be better if they did not have more children of their own, and she wanted to adopt a baby. Anne commented that, if Bob felt strongly about anything, it was impossible to change his mind; on this decision he was content to allow Anne to have her way.

For a while they did short-term fostering, and eventually they were told that a baby daughter awaited adoption. They had two days to make the practical preparations before they collected her; four months later she was legally their child.

With the two children the family was complete. Bob was always busy. As well as his work and his hobbies, he took courses in management and was promoted to a supervisory role in his firm. He enjoyed romping with the children when they were small, but did not like playing with them as much when they got older. However, he was conscientious in doing more structured activities with them. He took them to swimming lessons and, with their dog, they went to dog-training classes. When his son was old enough, he taught him to shoot and they went together to clay-pigeon shoots and wildfowling.

Bob built an extension in the roof for the children to use as a playroom and later he built a swimming-pool in the garden; when the family needed more space, he added a large extension to the bungalow. He and Anne enjoyed working in the garden together; they grew flowers and vegetables and had a large greenhouse.

He continued to be very cautious about money and had to be sure that he could pay for whatever he decided to build. Next, he built a boat and the family started sailing. He was very safety-conscious and would not take the family out in the boat until he felt confident about his own skill. They sailed on rivers; he never wanted to sail at sea. Anne said that she would have been happy to do things on the spur of the moment, even take the odd risk, but she had respect for her husband's caution and need for security.

During these years Bob had a lot of hobbies, some of which included the children and Anne, others of which did not. He played squash and badminton and took up golf. He always wanted to be competent at any sport. Although he got to know people through his hobbies, he made few friends and had no deep friendships. Anne commented that when she made a friend, that was a friend for life, but with Bob they came and went. He did not ask his friends home to eat; the people who did come to their home were her friends.

When the children were teenagers, Anne took responsibility for them. Bob lost interest but Anne needed to know where they were, with whom and what they were doing. During this time Bob and Anne might go out as many as five evenings a week together, although they both worked all day. They would have a family evening meal together and then go out, either for a sporting activity or to a dinner dance. They both enjoyed dressing up and the formality of ballroom dancing with live music.

After the children left home, Anne and Bob went on a series of adventurous holidays. They now had more money and no longer had any responsibility for elderly parents or dependent children. They shared a great enthusiasm for new things. Anne may have been the instigator, but Bob was, at first, happy to go along. They went on several holidays designed for eighteen- to thirty-year-olds, although Bob was by then over fifty. They took up skiing, canoeing and wet gliding then decided that they would take some long-haul holidays. They went to the USA and to New Zealand and their last big holiday was to Canada. They had plans to go to

Australia to see the Great Barrier Reef, but they did not manage that. After their return from Canada an event occurred that seems to have marked a turning point in Bob's life and health.

At the same time as Bob started to have more exotic holidays, his elder sister developed Parkinson's disease, from which she died three years later. She was married but had not been able to have children. She had been the strong one in her marriage, but during the last two years of her life, when her mind was failing as well as her body, and she was in a wheelchair, her husband looked after her. Bob regularly drove a long distance to bring his sister and her husband back to his home, so that her husband could have a short respite. But he was distressed by his sister's illness and did not want to speak about it. She died in a coma in hospital. Bob and Anne went to see her, but Bob was not able to touch her or sit with her because he wanted to get away too badly.

A few years later, his elder brother developed Alzheimer's disease and again Bob was unable to speak about his feelings. He did not like going to see his brother; after one visit he told Anne to be sure that he himself never got like that. He repeated the pattern of denying his feelings, keeping quiet and to himself. He wanted to blot out all thoughts and feelings about his sister and brother.

By 1985, Anne was aware that Bob was changing, although she says she had not thought about the possibility of his having Alzheimer's disease. If they were out with friends she noticed that he became like her shadow; he needed her there to answer any questions. Before, she considered that they had been independent of each other to a large degree. From that time, he started telephoning her from work. The telephone call would not be about anything in particular, but he would want to know if she was all right, or he would make a comment about retirement. He might ask her if she thought they could manage financially if he retired soon. She dismissed these calls as something trivial that would pass, but she still remembers them as surprising. Later she wondered if this could have been a moment for him to have spoken about his fears and feelings, but they had never shared deep anxieties, and at that time she made no attempt to change the pattern of their relationship.

Bob gradually gave up his hobbies and devoted nearly all his time and energy to his work. He no longer played golf because he said he could not find the time to practise enough and remain proficient. Anne thought that he was obsessed by his work, and began to feel resentful that he was neglecting her. She wonders now, more than ten years after these changes in Bob, if he had some awareness that his brain was failing, and felt that it was important to use all his energy to hang on to his work. He had been with the firm for most of his working life and it now became, apparently, his main object in living. He was responsible for big development projects and had to negotiate with and reprimand employees. He was always on call and had to cope with all kinds of emergencies. Other staff in his office realised that he was in some sort of difficulty and were supportive. With the benefit of hindsight, Anne thinks now that he was split in two. Half of him wanted to give up and ease the stress. There is evidence of that desire in his repeated questioning about whether they had enough money for him to retire, and his need for reassurance that they would be all right. But his life was intricately entwined with his firm, and his success in it and his pride prevented him from stating his own needs. He was not able to express his agony and Anne was not able to enter into it.

Anne remembers 1987 as a year of crises and difficulties. She was very ill early in that year. At first she was in bed at home, unable to get out of bed. Bob seemed to be in a panic and did not know what to do. He continued to go to work. Later she was in hospital and Bob set out to visit her. He did not arrive, and later said he had gone to the hospital but found that the ward was closed. Apparently he had gone to the wrong ward and had not asked for any information.

They had wanted to go to Canada for a considerable time, and later that year, when Anne was better, decided they would make the trip. But Bob appeared to have lost interest and showed no initiative. Anne made all the plans and Bob seemed content to go along with her decisions. The holiday was enjoyable for both of them, but Bob was unusually passive about everything. Bob had a new company car which they had taken to the airport. On their return, they collected it and were both relieved that it was still safe in the car park. Bob started the long drive home while Anne navigated. They took a wrong turn off the motorway and found a place where they could stop and look at the map. While they were pulled off the road and stationary, a large lorry crashed into the back of their car, pushing them forward. Bob showed no concern for Anne, but got out of the car and showed uncharacteristic, almost child-like fury with the lorry driver. Anne tried to calm him down. The lorry driver got out of his cab and apologised, explaining that he had not seen them. Bob was in a panic; Anne said that he flapped around.

Eventually the police arrived, arrangements were made for their car to be towed away, and Bob and Anne were taken to a small local cottage hospital by ambulance. It was Sunday morning, the casualty department was very quiet, and there was no doctor present. Bob became more agitated. He kept saying that he should not be there because he was all right; his main concern was for the car. Eventually a doctor arrived and checked them both over. Bob was given a neck support but Anne was all right.

They telephoned a member of the family to pick them up but Bob insisted that, before they could go home, he must go and see the car. He explained the urgency by saying that they must have their luggage. They found out where the car had been towed but, when they got there, the compound was locked and unattended. It had started raining heavily but Bob refused to abandon his search for the car and luggage and be driven home. Bob and Anne sat in silence in the back of the car and waited. They were both hungry, but Bob said that they could not go and get anything to eat or drink because the owner of the compound might come back and they would then lose the opportunity of checking the car and getting their luggage.

After two hours the men in charge of the compound did return, and they collected their luggage. They were then driven to the station and got a train home. Although Bob was clearly very shaken by the experience, he was back at work the next morning. This incident seems to have marked a turning point, both in his mental state and in Anne's understanding that there was indeed something amiss with him.

When Anne spoke about this incident, eight years later, she said that it had seemed at the time as though Bob was as much, or even more, damaged than the car. It was particularly important to him that it was the firm's car, and that it was new. Anne tried to say to him that a car was only a means of transport, something for getting from one place to another, but he could not accept that. She had never seen him in such a distraught state. He seemed to feel almost unbearably guilty; he worried that he would have to report the damage and also that he would be responsible for hiring a car for several weeks, until the damaged one was repaired. Anne felt that Bob was not in his normal state of mind; the amount of distress was out of proportion to the damage done either to him or to the car. It seemed to have an enormous and disastrous significance for him that could not be explained rationally. Anne kept trying to say to him, 'We're all right, aren't we?' and then she added, when she spoke with me, 'But we weren't'.

From then on, Bob found it more difficult to cope and became increasingly obsessed by his work. He had restless nights, would wake and write notes, and then get up at 5 am to go to work so that he could catch up with his paperwork before he was disturbed by the rest of the workforce. After his evening meal he went back to work, to check that everywhere was locked up and secure against a break-in. His life was work, sleeping and a minimum of food. He became absent-minded but his workmates were supportive. He struggled on for another three years which Anne thinks must have been very difficult years for him. One night during this time he got up to go to the bathroom, but he was unable to find the bedroom door. Bob said he felt as though his brain was going but Anne could find no way to speak with him about this fear. She did suggest that he should see a doctor, because she wondered if antidepressants might help him; but he rejected that suggestion. She made an appointment for him to go to their doctor, ostensibly to have an overdue tetanus immunisation. His doctor thought that he might have a depressive illness, but Bob refused to have any treatment.

The economic recession started in England in 1990, and Bob was offered early retirement. Anne knew that this was sensible, and also realised that it was a good way of release for his firm because, during the preceding years, he had needed much support from them; but Bob did not want to leave. It was clear that the work was causing him a lot of difficulty; he was spending longer hours achieving less, and his driving was erratic.

Retirement did give him some relief but Anne noticed that he always had an anxious look in his face. He kept the firm's car after he retired, but he never drove it again and the car stood in the drive. Anne had her own car and Bob would drive that.

Bob was brought up as Church of England but had no interest in the church. Anne had been brought up as a Methodist. She had always been connected with the church and her attachment had grown closer during the preceding years. After Bob's retirement he enjoyed going to church services with Anne because he liked singing.

Anne went on doing a little part-time work and would leave Bob his food and a list of jobs to do while she was out. At first he seemed to enjoy preparing the vegetables for the evening meal and digging in the garden. Anne started marking off the days on the calendar so that Bob did not lose touch with the day and month. Gradually he forgot to do the jobs and then forgot to eat the meals that Anne left ready for him.

One Sunday, early in 1993, Anne and Bob went out to lunch with friends near their home. Bob did not want to go out but agreed reluctantly. As soon as the meal was finished, he became anxious to get home. It was only a short walk, and they agreed that he would go and Anne would stay for coffee. She arrived home half an hour later but he was not there. She informed the police, but it was not until the next morning that he was found in a shed several miles away. It had been an extremely cold night and he was wearing a light coat. He had only survived because he had taken shelter in the shed. Ostensibly he had mistaken a turning and walked in the wrong direction but, interestingly, he had in fact walked to the area where he had lived as a child. Anne realised that he now needed her at home all the time and she gave up work straightaway.

Following this incident he went downhill more rapidly. Anne says that no diagnosis had been made, and Bob would not wait at the local hospital when he was sent there for investigation. Anne began to find it very difficult to keep him clean. He would not clean his teeth, wash himself, bath or shave. He refused all offers of help from Anne. Sometimes he would allow her to wash his feet in a bowl of water, but he seemed to have developed a fear of water. He would wear clean clothes, but his hair grew long and unkempt and he grew a beard. Eventually she asked for help, hoping to arrange for somebody to come to the house to bath him. To her surprise, it was arranged that Bob should be admitted to hospital for assessment and a trial of medication. He was in hospital for six weeks and after his discharge Anne had regular help at home. By this time he was incontinent, but the medication made him more easily manageable and he could be washed and shaved, dressed, undressed and put to bed more easily. From then on he has attended day care every weekday from 10 am until 3 pm and is admitted to hospital for a week every two months so that Anne can have a break and her own holiday.

Anne knows that the man she married has left her, and that now she is not his wife but his carer. There are still rare moments when something seems to get through to him and she catches a fleeting glimmer of the man he was. He has not talked for a long time but one day, shortly before we met, he belched and then said 'Pardon me'. Those words were a highlight, a brief moment of pleasure, for Anne. She describes him as, in most ways, a large and unresponsive baby. He must be changed, fed and dressed. He has tried to eat a domino and he bites the sheets when he is in bed. Anne says that it is possible to teach somebody, even in that state, ways of helping to be dressed; for example she holds up a sock and he raises a foot. But, she says sadly, you can't teach somebody to smile at you, and she longs for that more than for anything else. She remembers that once, long after he had stopped smiling, they were out for a slow walk and a dog barked. Bob gave a half-hearted smile. A dog came to stay for a weekend, but Bob ignored it and just shuffled past it. Anne explained that if she could get a smile she could feel that there was still a little bit of Bob inside the blankness. The rest of the time he was like an empty shell. She goes on hoping because it was a great thrill for her when he did smile, and it gave her a reminder of their former relationship. She added that a smile meant that there was some connection between two people.

When I listened to Anne telling me the story of her husband, I felt a great respect for her ability both to be committed to his care and to realise with clarity that the man she loved and married has gone and will not return. This enables her to help him as his 'carer', without sentimentality but with the necessary respect and feeling, and at the same time accept all the help she is offered. This gives her the opportunity to prepare herself for the next part of her own life, after his inevitable death.

I knew Anne before this encounter and guessed that she had these qualities. She is the only narrator I met who is actively caring for somebody with Alzheimer's disease. She was able to tell Bob's story clearly, without confusing it with her own story. She shows great courage, discipline and discrimination. Short of totally unforeseen circumstances, she will survive him to continue to live a creative life.

At one point, when Bob was already severely afflicted, she wrote out his story because she thought it would be interesting for his carers at the day centre and for their grandchildren. I believe this was an important step for her.

The meaning of money

During his last years at work, Bob repeatedly asked Anne if they had enough money for him to retire. It was such a constant theme that I have questioned its meaning. I have often heard a married woman say that she is short of money. This could literally be true, but on several occasions I have felt that she is uttering a doubt about her own worth as a person. Am I valuable in my own right or only as my husband's wife? Money is connected with the extrinsic value of a person and not with their innate worth which cannot be taken away. I wonder if, for Bob, the question, 'Do we have enough money so that I can retire?' could be translated into 'Am I of sufficient value to survive without the importance of my job?' I think he was concerned with establishing his value in the outer world rather than daring to search for it in the inner.

Problems and solutions

When Bob could not make the decision to give up work, he and Anne both used his work as the problem to be solved. Anne, at one level, blamed overwork for the change in him and thought that he would be better if he retired. Bob hung on to his work to try to stop the changes which he feared. They colluded in using work to maintain the *status quo*. My husband, John, did the same, and I colluded. He had to hang on to his work to give him his status and sense of value. I knew he was changing but thought that, if only he could give up his work, come back to me and his family, and fulfil his dreams, it would be all right. If work is the problem, the solution is to give it up or go on with it; but if work means status and value the visible problem is only the tip of an iceberg.

The damaged car

The car is a common theme through so many of these stories. The *Dictionary of Word Origins* gives the origin of the word 'car' as coming from a Latin word for two-wheeled chariot. It is probably linked with the words 'current' and 'course' with an underlying meaning of 'move swiftly'. The word 'career' is from the same origin, and originally meant 'a road or racetrack for vehicles'.

Bob's identification of himself with the new car is very strong; how else can we account for his irrational and unexpected behaviour when the car was hit by the lorry? Of course, such an incident is always shocking and distressing but for him, at that moment, it was of very great significance. Did he show more passionate feeling at that moment than ever in his life before? It is as though he saw himself as profoundly damaged. After his retirement he would never drive his car again, never get back into his own driver's seat, although for a time he did drive Anne's car.

People with Alzheimer's disease make great attempts to keep going, to hang on to the work which, until that time, has given their life a meaning. They also hate to give up their car, although they often drive recklessly and break rules. It is as though, driven by their failing reason, something forces them to fly in the face of danger. I think again of the legend of Icarus.

In symbolic language, the chariot represents the various parts of the human personality that are controlled by the charioteer, the driver. The charioteer is the representative of either the supreme god of reason, or the balance between reason and feeling. Can the driving force of reason lose touch with ordinary earthy things? Anything which loses touch with the earth will fall, and what falls from a height can break up.

CHAPTER 8

Maud

Maud's daughter, Gillian, told me that her mother is the third of four daughters of a well-established, intelligent and wealthy family from Chicago. Each year the family migrated to their summer home at Cape Cod, and it was while they were there that Maud was born in Boston. This marked her as a special person in the family because the other daughters were born in Chicago. Her father was of Scottish-Canadian origin, a brilliant and innovative scientist. His wife was born in Chicago to immensely wealthy parents who had made their money in industry. She must have been exceptionally intelligent and studied medicine at the University of Chicago. Every summer her family spent three months in their seaside home in the east and, on one of these occasions, she met her future husband. They were engaged in 1894 and, although she completed her medical training and qualified, she never practised.

Gillian has very fond memories of this grandmother, whom she saw as powerful, charismatic and extroverted. Gillian thinks that her grandmother saw her as a rather pathetic child who needed protection. Her grandmother had a great need to care for people and the small granddaughter filled her need. Gillian lived as a child in California with her parents, and her trips to the east were of immense importance to her. She remembers setting up an altar with her grandmother, who was a devoted Roman Catholic convert.

Before her grandmother's conversion to Catholicism she had toured Europe and had discussions with eminent Roman Catholics in London and Paris. Nobody else in the family converted and her husband was against the Catholic church. Gillian's mother, Maud, was the only one who seemed to have had any interest.

Gillian saw little of her beloved grandmother during the war years of 1939 to 1945. She thinks that travel during those years was too difficult for her to make the journey. Her grandmother was dementing, and Gillian knew that the family was concerned that she might give all her great wealth away to the Church. There were discussions about getting powers of attorney. By the time Gillian saw her grandmother again, there was a marked change. She had become very repetitive, but the disintegration never made her difficult, only more amusing. She was always able to live in the family home in Chicago and the summer home in Massachusetts. There were sufficient staff to care for her until her death in 1958. Her husband had died ten years earlier.

The grandmother's first baby was a boy who died. She was very distressed and adopted a baby boy. She then had two daughters of her own and then adopted another son, who was blind and played an important role in the future life of the family. The next baby was Maud and then, two and a half years later, there was another baby girl who died at the age of a few months in mysterious circumstances. The baby had been put on a bed for a sleep in a downstairs room and her mother had gone upstairs for a rest. A ten-year-old boy cousin, who was staying, had been naughty and, as a punishment, he was locked in the same room as the baby. The eldest sister, also ten years old, went into the room and found the baby dead, squashed between the bed and the wall. The boy cousin came to stay with the family again the following year, at Cape Cod; it is said that, while sleepwalking, he fell through an upstairs window and broke both his arms.

This was one of a number of events in this large family that was never talked about. It was as though all feelings were put under wraps. Grandmother had a serious depression and converted to Roman Catholicism. She built a clifftop shrine for the dead baby, and from then on became much involved in religion. Maud never spoke to her own family, including Gillian, about this tragedy; it was very much later that Gillian heard about it.

The grandfather was described as an honourable man, but he always had his own work and research and teaching, and withdrew to a large extent from his family. He was a Presbyterian, always taciturn and remote, a busy and important man, old-fashioned, with high standards,

Grandmother had a fourth and last daughter four years later; she was six years younger than Maud. An illiterate Irish nurse shared a room with the baby and Maud and brought them up. She was a warm-hearted Catholic. Many years later, after Maud was very confused, she recognised a photograph of this girl, but not one of her mother. This relationship was probably the warmest one of her childhood, but when she decided to start working hard at school, and that ideas were the most important things in her life, she shut herself away from the nursemaid and didn't want to see her. Gillian comments that now, in her dementia, she is surrounded by kindly young women who are all warm-hearted like the nursemaid, and from whom Maud is happy to receive much cuddling.

The eldest sister, her mother's favourite daughter, became a doctor and died an alcohol- and smoking-related

death in her seventies. The next sister, her father's favourite
and also a doctor, developed Alzheimer's disease. The
youngest sister became an artist and suffered from manic
depressive psychosis for many years.

Of the three adopted sons, only the blind one seems to
have been accepted and had a secure place in the family. As
a child, Maud had a close and probably warm relationship
with this brother, but at some point in early adolescence,
possibly after the brother had been sent away to a boarding
school for the blind, this relationship wilted. The boy's relationship was then closest with his younger, artistic sister. He
was a talented and accomplished pianist but, when his
interests were concentrated on jazz, the family disapproved.
After he married, and lived in New York with many artistic
friends, the disapproval continued.

Maud's relationship with this older, handicapped brother
must have been ambiguous. From an early age, she was left
in charge of him, to be his eyes and guide, and he became
dependent on her. For a small child this must have been a
burdensome responsibility.

Maud went to a day school in Chicago but did not enjoy
it and left at sixteen. She then spent a year in Europe, with
suitable chaperones, before going to Vassar. Again, like her
birth in Boston, this tour of Europe marked her out as
special. Gillian thinks that Maud was depressed before she
was sent away on this tour and she continued to have
episodes of depression throughout her life. Later it was
Gillian who helped her through the attacks.

From the time that Maud returned from Europe, her
mind seems to have been set on work. When she started at
university her sights were set on becoming a successful and
intellectual person. She seems to have seen this aspect of

herself as the one that was most important. She read English, German and Italian and, during her student days, made a translation of *Faust* which was put on as a dramatic production.

Maud's two older sisters were already succeeding in their chosen profession of medicine. She saw her importance first in having led her big brother around and, later, in her academic prowess. She seems to have done very well at university. She spent every summer vacation with the family in their summer home but was not very sociable. These times at the coast seem to have been very important to her. One of the memories which she could speak about with any clarity, late in her dementia, was the occasion when she swam out to the fishing nets in the bay and a young man swam to meet her from the opposite direction and they talked together. Maud christened him Leander. This passing relationship was evidently of immense importance to her. She was about nineteen at that time, overweight, good looking but not pretty. This apparently superficial relationship never developed, but it stayed with her throughout her life as an important fantasy, some sort of unfulfilled romantic idyll.

I look again at the myth of Hero and Leander while I am writing this account and can imagine that Maud's life was lived along the route of this myth. Leander, a young man of Abydos, on the Asian side of the Hellespont, would swim across the water every night to meet Hero. She guided him by holding up a torch. But one night he was drowned on his way across, and in despair she threw herself into the water and was also drowned. The boy Maud met at the nets, who has remained in her inner and unfulfilled life, disappeared. So, eventually, did Maud's integrity.

Maud always remained deeply attached to her family's

home in Massachusetts. Eventually she bought a house of her own in the same area to which she tried to come back every year. After she had become very confused, she still asked to go there. One summer, with much organisation, this was arranged. Helpers were hired at huge expense, but Maud did not even know that she was there. However, she has continued to think and speak about her house, saying that she is going there to stay with her mother and father. A few years ago, while she was staying there with Gillian and some of Gillian's children, there was a hurricane in which the old family home was totally wrecked and Maud's own cottage flooded; but Maud no longer recognised the family home.

Maud's first husband was very different from her idealised boyhood sweetheart. He was a musician, eight years older than Maud. She saw it as a wonderful romance but, on the eve of the wedding, he tried to get out of the marriage. However the wedding did take place, in Chicago, and she later told Gillian the hideous tale of her wedding night, of the blood and the hurt. After the wedding they drove three thousand or so miles across the USA. Maud told Gillian of the horrors of the journey, of how she was left alone in the car while he went off and of how he mocked her. Maud described him to her daughter as a sadist. Gillian was born a year later and a younger brother five years after that. The marriage was near breakdown, but Maud wanted to conceive a second child before the divorce because she did not think it was a good thing for a child not to have a brother or sister.

Gillian describes her father as charismatic, like her grandmother, and she does not remember him saying a cross word. Maud divorced him because he was totally unreliable and she knew there were other women. He was charming, but insisted that he always had his own way. He remarried three times. He told Gillian, much later, that he never wanted a divorce and that he had loved all of his wives. Each one of them, in different ways, fell apart after their relationship with him and the inevitable divorce. His fourth wife was forty years younger than he. Maud told Gillian that she had married him because she found him romantic. She enjoyed writing poetry and he said that he would set it to music, though this did not happen.

Maud remarried and, with her own money, was able to set herself and her new husband up in a beautiful house. In this house she had her own study and typewriter and she decided to make a new translation of Dante's *Divine Comedy*. Her second husband was always able to make her think she was a wonderful woman, and he would allow nobody to criticise her.

Gillian was in early adolescence and had just started at a new school. She and some of her schoolfriends were walking past her home. Maud came out and wanted to join them, but Gillian said that she could not because she was too old. Maud was extremely distressed. Her husband arrived and asked Gillian, on her return, what on earth she had done to her mother. Maud lay and sobbed and did not speak while her husband stood over Gillian and administered justice. Gillian was threatened with being sent away to live with her real father, whom she hardly knew. Gillian now thinks that her mother's remarkable behaviour had a lot to do with her fear of old age. Being called 'old' by her teenage daughter precipitated this reaction. Maud, with her two older husbands, seems to have had fantasies of always being the small girl, dependent on a strong father. But both times she married men who were weak, charming and unreliable, the opposite of the strong man she was searching for.

The second husband was fourteen years older than Maud. He had a small war-service pension, but although he had contacts among the artistic people of San Francisco, he did very little. He did some writing and painting but never created any finished work.

Maud's second husband died in 1958, the same year as her mother. By this time Gillian was married and living in England. Her mother paid for her and the family to fly first class to stay with her in California. Gillian found this very hard and tiring, but her mother was convinced that she was providing a treat. She insisted that they stay for three or four weeks and, reluctantly, this is what Gillian did. She wonders now if her mother was not trying to buy love or attempting to repair a relationship which had probably never taken root.

After her second husband's death, Maud started teaching history in a Catholic school because she felt that she must 'do' something. She enjoyed meeting teachers and parents and became very friendly with some of the nuns. During this time she started to have strong friendships with other women, particularly with one younger woman. This young woman, who appointed herself Maud's companion, introduced her to a younger man who was very charismatic and seemed to have *bona fide* publishing contacts. Maud was now seventy-five years old and he was thirty years younger, married and with children. He persuaded Maud to rewrite her autobiography, which she had written earlier. He wanted to get it illustrated and arrange for it to be published.

Maud abandoned all her good works and devoted herself to this young man. She agreed to pay for all his credit-card expenses and he escorted her on extensive European tours. Then he arranged for her to move into a retirement home, having first sold her own house to raise the money, and Maud seemed delighted to allow him to manage all her affairs. She did not have a lawyer or an accountant and her mind was getting vague. Maud's children and grandchildren did not see any of the money raised by the house sale.

She was still driving in the late 1980s, but got lost driving a route on the east coast which she knew very well. She decided that it was not safe to go on and telephoned a young relative to ask for help, but when he arrived to fetch her she had forgotten that she had asked for help. She became disturbed, and felt threatened by his appearance and his expectation that she would get into his car.

In 1991 she had abdominal pain and went into hospital for an exploratory operation. After the operation she had pneumonia and suddenly her dementia got worse. She started wandering away from her apartment at night and making many telephone calls to her companion and her son with requests that they tell her where she was. The young man disappeared from the scene about this time, and Maud appeared to forget about him. She was moved to the medical floor of the retirement home.

The retirement complex was no longer suitable for the care of a woman who was dementing. Her companion attempted to organise and control her care by bringing in therapists of various sorts to improve her state of mind. Maud's son, who lived close by, did not want to get too involved with his mother, possibly fearing her more in her present state than he had earlier in life, when she seemed to be in charge of her own destiny. If she left the retirement complex, a considerable sum of her capital would be lost, and this influenced the decision-making. The companion was paid to keep an eye on her, visit her regularly and generally supervise her care and comfort. Eventually the situation became too confused and her son stepped in and took control. The companion was dismissed and Maud was moved to a nursing home which catered for the mentally confused.

An empty shell

Gillian goes to see her mother when possible, but Maud no longer knows her. She occasionally telephones, but her mother now has no understandable speech. Gillian describes her as an empty shell. It is strange to look at this woman from a distance and attempt to see who or what she is. Although I spent many hours listening to her daughter and am well aware of the enormous influence she has had on her, I am left with little real knowledge of the person that was Maud; and this is strongly reminiscent of Amanda. I had no idea, before starting this search across the Atlantic, of any similarities between these two stories. In some ways their narratives are very different. Maud comes from an immensely privileged background, in terms of money, property, social establishment and education. During the telling of her story, Gillian on various occasions spoke of the details that gave Maud a sense of being special. Being in the middle of so many children, natural and adopted, and the third of four daughters, she must have needed ways of establishing that she was indeed special and unique. The first was the place of her birth. She was born in Boston but the other daughters were born in Chicago. During her early childhood she was special because she was the guide for her blind older brother.

This role must have given her remarkable power at an extra-ordinarily early age over another human being, a handi-capped male, as well as many demanding responsibilities for so young a girl. In the telling of her story, the sense of com-mitment and responsibility and the resulting importance was clear; but I did not hear any sense of warmth or tenderness or strong feeling. These were reserved for the nursemaid. Maud seems to have been prepared to let go of her respon-sibility with alacrity when the brother was sent to boarding school; and this separation was final when she did her tour of Europe. She had contempt for his jazz and did not have any ongoing relationship with him or his wife. The youngest sister picked up this relationship at the point where Maud abandoned it, but it was a very different sort of relationship. She enjoyed his music, and they had their artistic talents in common.

The dead baby image

The recurrent theme of the dead baby seems to fall like a shadow over the person who dements. A dead baby boy is a very powerful image hanging over a small replacement girl. The dead boy has a great and invisible power. No living child can aspire to that level of perfection. I heard the same theme in the story of Elspeth. The girls who have grown up under this overwhelming, dark shadow seem to marry men who are inferior to them. They are shorter, not as wealthy, of lower social standing, less clever or with a touch of the reprobate. Is it to achieve some sort of balance between the supremely good, dead, male to which they cannot aspire that they find a mate whom they can, in turn, overshadow? Of course, they would not be aware of this, but I wonder if it is an underlying recurrent pattern that I have seen in Amanda, Elspeth and now in Maud. It begins to look like the same thread of fate.

Other common themes

Maud, in common with Elspeth, Amanda, John and Alice needed, at an early age, to find a secure and controllable place for herself. For differing reasons, they were not in a warm and accepting emotional climate in which they could develop in a balanced way. It looks as though an early chill factor has pushed them into the position of having to control and dominate their own destinies. Trust and acceptance were in short supply for these people early in their lives. Their safe place was in intellectual achievement and in the outer appurtenances of life, attractive homes, clothes and money. They all found it difficult to accept and mourn losses and to express strong feelings whether of joy or sorrow.

CHAPTER 9

Is there a common denominator?

I look and look again at the six narratives of the people who disintegrated. I want to look at 'stills' from their lives and try to understand if there are any pivotal moments which give a key to the underlying meaning of their break-up. First I have to choose a precise moment in the narrative, one which has struck the narrator with its importance. Then I need to be prepared to stay with this incident, picture it as vividly as I can, while I am in a place of quiet and stillness. It is a bit like moving out of the stream of traffic on the motorway into the central reservation. The traffic goes on but I am temporarily disengaged. To stay with each of these moments, I must be prepared to suspend my medical knowledge and scientific outlook. Each moment has passed and I know that I can change nothing. I want to make an attempt to appreciate the essence of the people involved and the relationship, or lack of relationship, between them, beyond the superficialities of dress and surroundings. These important, pivotal moments were a recurrent theme in the narratives: Bob and Anne and the damaged car; Maud's near-paralytic fury with her daughter at the idea that she was old; John, and the moment when he slammed the door on the possibility of relationship. From that time it seemed that a piece of him had moved out and he began to act like a boat without a rudder or an empty shell. Can the centre of a person become displaced?

While I sit in my quiet central reservation, I look at

Picasso's picture 'The Tragedy'. It is from his 'blue period' and is also titled 'Poor People on the Seashore'. The picture is of a man, a woman and a young boy. Although they are standing near each other, there is no sense of any relationship. The man and the woman appear sunk in their own separate worlds of tragedy, with downcast eyes, and their arms folded so that their hands are invisible. The boy's eyes are also out of contact with the viewer or the other characters, but his hands are visible. With his right hand, it looks as though he could be pushing his father away and, with his left, he could be making a gesture of supplication to his mother. I am supposing that the two adults are his mother and father, but there is nothing in the painting, apart from their proximity, to suggest the truth of such a supposition. There is no relationship. The painting of the figures and of the background is in blue. Although it is possible to distinguish the sky from the sea, and the sea from the beach, there are no clear boundaries and they appear to run into each other. There is no shelter. I am looking at a reproduction of this painting while I write. I see and imagine what I see; another person who spends time looking at the same painting will have her own reactions and they will almost certainly be different from mine. That is the nature of art; it is the response of the individual who is looking that is important. William Blake said that he did not see with his eyes but through his eyes; that is the seeing which happens while I sit quietly in this isolated central reservation of the motorway and look at the incidents in the narrations.

As I look at these six people, and at the narrators, I begin to see that there are common denominators across two continents, across class and sex and background. I begin to see strange similarities in the pattern. Going back to the Picasso picture, I wonder if this scenario, or a similar one, could be the setting which makes somebody prone to disintegrate; on the beach, without clear boundaries or any home, without an identified and named place, without the identifiable presence of a mother and a father.

Now I want to see the opposite face of that desolation. I take a photograph of a baby of two months, with his father and mother. The mother is holding the baby firmly, but in such a way that he is at her arm's length and can see her face. There is eye-to-eye contact between the mother and the child. The mother is sitting down and the child is supported on her lap. The father is standing about a foot behind the chair. He is watching both of them, standing over and protecting them, but not touching either of them. There is a great sense of relationship and joy in this picture.

I think of the moment when Gillian told Maud that she was too old to join her and her new schoolfriends on their walk. Her comment was the trigger for the scene I want to look at. After the walk, Gillian returned home and found her mother prostrate on a bed, with her new, older husband, who in many ways was dependent on her, standing over her. He disciplined Gillian, threatening to send her away to her natural father. Maud lay in a collapsed condition and said nothing. It is a moment of extraordinary desolation and pain. The natural father was absent, and a stand-in was acting the part. Maud absented herself, through her state of collapse, and was not able to take any responsibility for what was going on. Gillian was horrified and bewildered by the whole incident. I see the parallels here with the Picasso painting. The child, here Gillian, is not responsible for her own destiny at this moment. In order to survive, she must fall into the role of mediator. Her remark triggered the incident, but it was not intended to harm; she made it to defend her own insecure place in her society. Maud is both mother and wife, but she has opted out. The man goes through a ritual anger but it looks as though he is placating his wife. He never wants her to be criticised. Earlier incidents in Maud's life show that one way she established her specialness was to be the guide of her dependent, older, blind, adopted brother. From her teenage years she fell into a state of depression many times. Was this a means, not conscious or deliberate of course, of escaping from stressful situations? Of removing herself emotionally from times of loss and failure?

Then I look again at the damaged family, and the need of the child to protect itself from hurt as best it may, to suppress the feelings that are too painful to be borne. Could the pattern of alienation and dried-up desolation be passed on through the generations? Those who see the unhappiness will make attempts to change the pattern, and their destiny, by being more intellectually able or wealthier or having larger and more beautiful houses, but perhaps it cannot be changed in this way. The three blue people on the bare beach cannot be made better and happier in any superficial way.

I believe that all six people whose stories are told here were exceptionally head-bound people, controllers and organisers. Why are they like this? Each of them has been born into a family where they have been vulnerable, where feelings have been dangerous and threatening, and each has built some inner and inaccessible fortress in order to survive.

The inner and outer realities

During the past two hundred years or so there has been, in

the developed world, an explosion in man's understanding of himself and his mind and body, and also of the world around him. In the preceding two hundred years the foundations for this explosion were laid. Galileo, the Italian mathematician and astronomer, developed formulae to work out the laws of motion. With the aid of a telescope he examined the sky and confirmed Copernicus' view that the earth moved around the sun, and that the earth was not the centre of the universe as the Church then believed. He was brought before the Inquisition and forced to recant the evidence which he had seen through his own eyes. Irrational belief triumphed over rational knowledge.

The words 'rational' and 'reason' both come from the Latin word *ratio* which is derived from the verb *reri*, to reckon or calculate. 'Irrational' means 'not being endowed with reason, illogical, absurd'. Is there a possibility that a man can be both rational and reasoning at one level and, at another level, irrational and able to accept things which are not accessible to his reasoning powers? Sir Isaac Newton, the British mathematician and physicist, was born in 1642, the year in which Galileo died. He discovered the laws of gravity and of planetary motion, invented the calculus, and discovered that white light could be split into its constituent colours. He used his great rational powers to remarkable effect. However, in later life he became a recluse, and spent much time, day and night, in the study and practice of alchemy. He did not make public his interests in this field during his lifetime, but left many unpublished papers, discovered after his death, which confirm his interest.

Alchemy is a strange blend of chemistry and magic or mysticism. It originated in China and Egypt, probably about the same time, before the third century BC, and it spread through Asia and Europe, playing a part in both Islam and Christianity. Alchemy has a double meaning and interpretation, one in outer reality and the other in inner reality. At the outer level, the aim was to produce gold from base metals. This transformation was to be brought about through a long series of exact, measurable and disciplined physical processes. There was also the desire to produce an elixir which would give everlasting life, and a panacea for all the sicknesses of mankind. Alchemy was always a secret process, its methods known only to its initiates. However, underlying the outer reality, and the physical work with all its remarkable apparatus, there was always a different and inner meaning, the transformation of the alchemist's soul. The base metals were the whole of his body, mind and spirit, and the sum total of his life's experiences. The transformation could be brought about through the gathering together of all these disparate bits and the jettisoning of those that were not of any ultimate value. The inner work was long and arduous and required constant awareness and discrimination. The hope was for transformation into a unique and inner treasure, known only to the worker and his creator. The aim of the work was the finding of the lapis, or Philosopher's Stone.

Here is an Indian story which illustrates what I am trying to describe. Each day, the king sat in state hearing petitions and dispensing justice. Each day a holy man, dressed in the robe of an ascetic beggar, approached the king and, without a word, offered him a piece of very ripe fruit. Each day the king accepted the 'present' from the beggar and, without a thought, handed it to his treasurer who stood behind the throne. Each day the beggar, again without a word, withdrew and vanished into the crowd.

Year after year, this ritual occurred every day the king sat in office. Then one day, some ten years after the holy man first appeared, something different happened. A tame monkey, having escaped from the women's apartments in the inner palace, came bounding into the hall and leaped up onto the arm of the king's throne. The ascetic beggar had just presented the king with his usual gift of fruit, but this time, instead of passing it on to his treasurer as was his usual custom, the king handed it over to his monkey. When the animal bit into it, a precious jewel dropped out and fell to the floor.

The king was amazed and quickly turned to his treasurer behind him. 'What has become of all the others?' he asked. But the treasurer had no answer. Over all the years he had simply thrown the unimpressive 'gifts' through a small upper window in the treasure house, not even bothering to unlock the door. So he excused himself and ran quickly to the vault. He opened it and hurried to the area beneath the little window. There, on the floor, lay a mass of rotten fruit in various stages of decay. But amidst the garbage of many years lay a heap of precious gems.

Alchemy, as a way of producing gold in outer reality, can be and was dismissed as a lot of rubbish and outdated magic. From the time of Newton, man dispossessed himself of this sort of mystery which he saw as undesirable superstition. Newton lived to the good age of eighty-five. We can surmise that the scientific first half of his life and his public writing and teaching were in balance with the secret second half of his life, taken up with mystery and his personal and secret inner reality, his private preparation for his death. In the years after Newton's death, alchemy was relegated to the realms of outdated mediaeval life. It was seen as rotten fruit, of no immediate use and importance, and thrown away.

Carl Jung, in the course of his life and work, studied alchemy, not as a means of making gold in outer reality, but as a way of making sense of dreams in his own inner reality. Later, this understanding contributed to his work with those who came to him for help. Many of the symbols used by the alchemists are present in the dreams of those living at the end of the twentieth century.

Telescopes became more powerful and man could explore the great spaces around him, and with the help of microscopes could discover the minutiae of the constituent cells of his body, and the shape of the germs which attack him and cause illnesses. With inoculations and immunisations, he began to control these diseases. He discovered ways of using anaesthetic drugs to control pain, and surgical operations could then be more widely practised and were more acceptable to patients. In the nineteenth century, in Britain, Sir Edwin Chadwick promoted widespread public-health measures that provided clean water to drink and effective methods for the safe disposal of sewage. These measures were effective in controlling the spread of illnesses such as typhoid and cholera. In this century, scientists have put men on the moon and, at the time of writing this book, they are contemplating the possibility of putting hotels and developing tourism in outer space. Man, by the use of his conscious mind during these centuries, has developed a remarkable degree of control over his own body and over the world around him.

In the twentieth-century developed world, from the time that a child gives up playing, he lives in a world where he must learn to develop his mind and his body so that he can follow in this tradition of control in order to survive. The majority of men and women now live in a market-place for learning, and for getting and keeping control of themselves, their relationships and surroundings. The child has to become the person who can live in the family and society. This may bear little resemblance to the person he was created, but is the person he must be in order to cope with everyday life. Otherwise he will become an unacceptable misfit.

In the series of roles which we play, we are reliving Shakespeare's lines in *As You Like It*. 'All the world's a stage and all the men and women merely players: they have their exits and their entrances; and one man in his time plays many parts.' Shakespeare describes the parts or roles as inevitable stages in a man's life, ending with 'the lean and slipper'd pantaloon and finally to second childishness and mere oblivion'. Here there is a description of the return to a more passive stage at the end of life. In the modern world, much emphasis is put on the achievements of the first half of life, and much less on the inevitability of loss, of many kinds, in the second half of life.

In outer reality, during the first half of our lives we use our consciousness to learn the skills to survive and make a place for ourselves. It is the time, necessarily so, for getting qualifications and skills and achieving a recognisable place in society. There is a normal and socially acceptable progress from school to other training, to a profession or other paid employment, to meeting a mate, finding a home and possibly to having a family. Certainly many of those possibilities and likelihoods are changing at the end of the twentieth century, with more unemployment and frequent breakdown in marriage. However, it remains the time of defining our lives by what we have and what we do, not by who or what we are.

In Eric Fromm's book, *To Have or To Be*, there is an illuminating account of the different modes of living in the first and second halves of life, with some explanation of the predominance of the 'having' mode in Western society, which is commonly continued from the first half into the second part of life. Some of our possessions, such as our homes, cars, pets and books are easily identifiable. My home, my husband and my children are easily recognisable to myself, and to those around me, and they become extensions of myself in my personal outer reality. Possessions can go beyond this to include my health, my illness and my personal problems. Having health, or illness, as a possession is more easily understood than the state of being healthy or being sick, in a society which is geared to the 'having' mode. Possessions can be acquired and, by the same understanding, they can be disposed of; the owner can be dispossessed. Dementia can be more easily accepted as 'having Alzheimer's disease' than being in a state of disintegration. The disease can then be identified as something extraneous to the person who has it, and understood as an unwanted possession. Disease, once it is diagnosed, is the responsibility of the doctor, who should be able to take it away. If he is not able to do that yet, more scientific research will make it possible soon. More money will speed up the scientific advances. In a society which pays so much attention to the outer reality, this is the normal way to see disease.

During the centuries of the rapid development of man's conscious understanding and control of his outer reality, there has been a reciprocal denial of the importance of his inner reality. Our mediaeval ancestors certainly believed in a highly structured inner reality, with devils and angels and the hierarchy of heaven, earth and hell. Dante, in *The Divine*

Comedy, gives an extraordinary picture of a different understanding of the world, where the inner reality is balanced and
interconnected with the outer reality. The outer world of
the politics of Italy is balanced by the inner world of the
struggle of the powers of good and evil, of sins and virtues.

Roots and branches

The words 'conscious' and 'unconscious' have many meanings in the late twentieth century. In *Webster's Medical
Dictionary* 'conscious' is defined as '1. capable of or marked
by thought, will, design or perception . . . 2. having mental
faculties undulled by sleep, faintness or stupor'. In the same
dictionary 'unconsciousness' is defined as 'the greater part of
the psychic apparatus accumulated through life experience
that is not normally integrated or available to consciousness
yet is manifested as a powerful motive force in overt behaviour especially in neurosis and is often revealed as through
dreams, slips of the tongue'. There are those things in our
outer reality of which we are aware and those things of
which we are unaware.

During the last two centuries the words 'conscious' and
'unconscious' have been connected with various schools of
psychology. I want here to find a way of describing the disintegrating sickness of modern man without using these
words. If I imagine man as a tree, he has the visible parts, the
trunk and branches, above ground in the light, which I can
see with my eyes, and the invisible parts, the root system, in
the dark, invisible to my eyes but of which I can become
aware through my imagination. This is not a scientific
description, but picture language, dream language. The root

system of a tree, and of trees growing together in woodland, could be like the root system of humanity, as individual humans and as groups in families and societies. You cannot see, either literally or by reason, the roots of humanity any more than you can see the roots of a tree but it may be that humanity cannot survive in its fullness without healthy roots any more than can a tree.

'Aware,' in the *Dictionary of Word Origins* is derived from the word 'ware'. 'The prehistoric Germanic base *war*, *wer*, denoted watch, be on one's guard, take care and also produced English ward and warn. It may have had links with Latin *vereri*, fear (source of English revere). From it was formed the adjective *waraz*, which evolved into English ware, now virtually obsolete except in the derived forms aware, beware and wary.'

There are things in our outer and inner realities of which we are aware; and there are also things of which we are unaware. For example, while I am sitting at my desk writing I see the keyboard in front of me and I hear the clicking sounds as I press the keys. But there are many things around me, both in the realms of vision and hearing, of which for most of the time I am unaware. There is a desk lamp in front of me, an open door on the left, piles of papers and books on the desk. But until I allow my mind to move sideways and around I remain unaware of these things because my mind is directed towards the present goal, which is putting thoughts into words and onto paper. The same is true of hearing. There is a background noise of humming from the computer, some intermittent cracking sounds from the radiators and the howling of wind outside, but again these sound are peripheral to my present focus of attention.

There are triggers which can make us more aware of

things of which we have previously been unaware. A signal or warning can make us more alert. At this moment I am using my central vision while I look straight ahead. I am thinking, my mind is concentrated; but I can be alerted through vision or hearing to something beyond. For example, a sudden noise of birds from the garden alerts me to a prowling cat. My vision follows my hearing, I see the marauder and can then go and take action, or decide to allow nature to take its course. This is a simple example of the inborn alert system which, at this level, works through my sensory organs. Provided I am capable of being aware, I can choose whether I take action or do not take action. This is part of the alert system at the visible tree level; but there is another alert system which operates from root level.

Root disease or genetic inheritance?

Genetic disease is inherited from one generation to another in a recognisable pattern. The genetic inheritance of any disease is a matter built into the physical body. It is not under the control of the owner, who has no choice over whether the condition will be manifest or not. There is always the hope and possibility that one day it may be scientifically possible for changes to be carried out on the genes. However, if one looks at the ways in which family traits are inherited, beyond what is physical and measurable in genes, I postulate that inheritance may occur through the root system of mankind. In one sense, we are all interconnected. In another sense, we have the free will, if we dare, to look at what is happening, and we then have the potential to work differently with the raw materials of our lives. I believe that patterns of behaviour in families hold the potential for change.

If there were conditions of sickness in the root system of mankind, they would be in the dark and hidden; we would not be able to see them nor measure them nor understand how to control them. They would be incomprehensible in the clear and uncomplicated light of man's reason. Reason depends on the abstract word and idea; 'abstract' is described in the *Shorter Oxford English Dictionary* as derived from 'Latin *abs* away and *trahere* draw. Separated from matter, practice or particulars.' Man, through his power to think and organise, has most control over his outer reality. If a tree has no roots, or it is cut like a Christmas tree, it lasts only a short time and then inevitably withers and dies. Without roots it has lost its sources of food and drink.

The custom of having a Christmas tree decorated with lights, with presents beneath it, probably is derived from a tree of Norse mythology. Yggdrasil was the world tree, and its roots and branches represented heaven, earth and hell. It is a feature of the Icelandic myth of creation, in which the earth is represented as a circle of land with the ocean around. In the middle of the earth is the tree, and its roots go down into the underworld, which is a source of wisdom. At the root lies a serpent, in the top branches is an eagle, and a squirrel runs up from the roots to the branches taking messages and sewing strife.

Just as there are triggers which alert us to new things, good or bad, in the periphery of our outer reality, are there comparable triggers, some sort of squirrel, in our inner reality, which can deliver messages from the individual or shared depths of man? In the internal and invisible anatomy of man, how can the squirrel be identified? How can the messages between the serpent in the depths and the eagle in its look-out position at the top of the tree be decoded?

This concept is getting into the level of a dream world, and dreams are the messages from the root system. Dreams have been described as secret letters from my self, the inmost, most secret, most awe-inspiring piece of me, that cannot be seen or measured or known, and is not open to scientific investigation. Some physical and mental symptoms, illnesses, weaknesses, failures and losses could also be part of the squirrel alert system from the root level within each individual. In the Icelandic myth of Yggdrasil, the messages of the squirrel can cause war between the serpent and the eagle, destruction as well as creation. Some of these symptoms could be private messages about our own lives and mortality. The threats of death, the losses of control, could be welcomed as guidance; but if they become illnesses to be taken away and cured, they are denied. They can then be of no possible benefit to the person. We say, 'Doctor take it away, make me better.' The illness is put in the wastepaper basket and is no longer of any value. I believe there is an alternative way, of acceptance of the whole of one's self, that can lead to a more creative old age.

Symbols

The word 'symbol' is defined in the *Dictionary of Word Origins* as meaning 'something thrown together'. From it was derived a word meaning 'identifying token' and that meant an outward sign of something. A dream is the surest way of hearing the alerts from deep in the root system. The symbols in the dream throw one world into the other, roots into branches, serpent into eagle, acting as a mysterious adhesive which holds the two levels together; but the line of demarcation is clear and there is no confusion between the levels. *The Shorter Oxford English Dictionary* defines 'symbol' as 'something that stands for, represents, or denotes something else (not by exact resemblance, but by vague suggestion, or by some accidental or conventional relation); especially a material object representing or taken to represent something immaterial or abstract. Symbol can also be an object representing something sacred.'

Fire was used by the alchemists to keep their retorts burning at exactly the right temperature to transform base metals into gold. If the fire lost too much heat, or went out, the work would be wasted and the whole process had to be started again. If the fire flared up and got too hot, the transformation would be ruined and, again, many months of work might be lost. Of course, everybody with any intelligence, at the end of the twentieth century, knows all that is rubbish. Certainly it is at the outer level. But fire, as a visible and concrete thing at the outer level, could also have another meaning at the inner level. Anybody who is involved in any creative activity knows that daily return to that activity is necessary, whether it is writing or potting or playing a musical instrument. If you miss many days of work at your artistic skill, your ability falls off. If you try to accelerate the performance of your skill by working for too many hours without a break, you can collapse under the strain. Here the fire is not the literal sort, made of coal and wood and lit by a match, but the fire of discipline, commitment and concentration.

The symbols that are presented in dreams have opposite meanings. Fire can either be a way of cooking, warming and purifying or, if allowed to get out of control, can burn and destroy. In a similar way water is either a fountain or river, a source of life; or the opposite, a deluge or flood which destroys and eliminates life.

Personal and individual symbols are presented to us in dreams and can be of people, water, bridges, ladders, numbers, colour and animals. They can be houses, rooms in houses, and many others. Many symbols go back far beyond the individual to ancient Egyptian, Greek and Christian mythology and symbolism. The symbols that occur in dreams cannot be interpreted in the ways of outer reality because symbols are the language of the inner reality, a different language.

The key is a symbol which has had meaning through thousands of years in many religions, including Christianity. At the level of outer reality it is used for the opening and closing of doors, locking and unlocking, making safe and releasing to freedom. It is the token of St Peter and also of a gaoler. A key has clear and opposite meanings, like water and fire. When I went to John's flat, I found several locks on the front door, two spy holes and a chain. The keys and locks could be a means of attempting to keep a secure boundary, a demarcation line, between him and some inner chaos that was overwhelming him. The chaos was at the inner level but the boundaries were inappropriate because they were made at the outer level.

A bridge in dream, poetry or a painting, is frequently a symbol of a change or transition. It can be from one place to another, or from life to death. Again, we have to realise that the meaning in the dream cannot be interpreted in the literal way of outer reality, because in the inner reality there are always the opposite meanings. An old lady listened to a lecture on William Blake. She looked at one of his illustrations in *Songs of Experience*; it was a picture of London with a child leading an old man through a door. She asked the lecturer where they were going to. She wanted to know which way was in and which way was out. Was the child leading the old man to something good or bad? The lecturer continued talking, but the questions recurred. Clearly the woman found the picture of great significance and she wanted clear answers to her questions. She had no feeling about making her own interpretation. A door symbolises a way through, out or in. In a dream, the dreamer must find out what the interpretation is for himself and at that particular time. A closed door might be a hidden mystery, and an open door an opportunity for a different way ahead and the possibility of freedom.

A house can be a symbol of the inner home, the safe place, in a dream. We all need an outer safe place but when we are in a state of emotional balance we do not confuse our inner and outer realities. The wanderings, particularly at night, of those who are disintegrating do, I think, represent this search for their home, but the level is confused. At moments of anxiety there is an instinct in most of us to be at home. Two friends have, in the past two days, told me of recent illnesses, when they have been well cared for by relatives but had an urgent need to return home in order to make a full recovery. This instinct is strong and good as long as the levels do not get mixed.

Boundaries

In outer reality, most of us have an instinct about how close we like to be to somebody else. The London Underground at rush hour can strain that instinct to its uttermost limits in many of us. Some people do not seem to have an instinct about what is an acceptable distance between people. They get too close during a conversation and then a person who does know her boundaries instinctively moves away. In the use of language, the French observe very clear boundaries between people. *Madame* and *Monsieur* are the acceptable manner of address until you know somebody well, and they do not rush into the use of Christian names. *Tu* is used in families and amongst close friends and to children but otherwise there is the more formal *vous*. These differences denote degrees of relationship and define some of the minutiae of boundaries between people.

Ostensibly at the outer level, Robert Frost writes in a poem 'Good fences make good neighbours'. Boundary disputes are a very common and distressing cause of conflict between neighbours and of war between countries. However, we do not want our boundary fences or our customs posts at international frontiers to be so thick, high and impenetrable that we may never meet or relate to our neighbours. We need the discipline of good boundaries in order to exercise the choice of when we make a connection with the neighbour on the other side. Without a boundary there will be total confusion and war.

At an inner level, boundaries are equally important, but the necessary boundaries here are more difficult to describe because they are not apparent to our eyes. The essential boundary is between the personal, deep, secret inner reality and the outer reality. These boundaries must not be so impenetrable that the person in his outer reality knows nothing of what is happening in his inner reality. If they are, such a person is then separated from his own meaning and lacks the nourishment to live a full life. The interconnection between the inner and outer realities is more necessary as he gets older, because it is part of the transition from his active doing and achieving time to his more passive and receptive period.

Boundaries are not only a necessary part of our personal inner and outer realities, and between our neighbours, but they are also an essential part of all the creation myths of the world. In the Judaeo-Christian tradition, the book of Genesis describes with clarity the laying out and defining of these boundaries. From the beginning of Chapter 1:

In the beginning God created the heaven and the earth. And the earth was without form, and void; and darkness was upon the face of the deep. And the Spirit of God moved upon the face of the waters. And God said, 'Let there be light': and there was light. And God saw the light, that it was good: and God divided the light from the darkness. And God called the light Day, and the darkness he called Night. And the darkness and the light, the day and night were distinct from each other and each had its boundaries. And God said, 'Let there be a firmament in the midst of the waters, and let it divide the waters from the waters.' And God made the firmament, and divided the waters which were under the firmament from the waters which were above the firmament: and it was so. And God called the firmament Heaven . . . And God said, 'Let the waters under the heaven be gathered together unto one place, and let the dry land appear.' And it was so. And God called the dry land Earth; and the gathering together of the waters called he Seas.

I do not suggest that we need to believe in the literal story of the creation in seven days, but it has great mythological meaning for the understanding of our personal lives. A person who has lived life in the outer reality with some success, and who has paid no attention to his inner world, where the boundaries between his personal inner and outer realities have become so dense and impenetrable, seems to be particularly prone, at the onset of dementia, to a breakdown in those boundaries. From the outside these can be seen as bizarre occurrences, possibly minor criminal acts, such as driving offences, or social infringements; but they are all done without the conscious awareness or any responsibility on the part of the disintegrating person. It is as though there has been a build-up of pressure behind a dam. Then something makes the dam burst and totally unexpected things happen.

An old lady, who was without family or friends, lived a solitary life. Over the course of many years she had made a number of hostile relationships. One day, she employed a man to knock down a fence between herself and one neighbour, and severely damage an old holly hedge between herself and her other neighbour. She then spent a great deal of time peering through the gaps in the damaged boundaries. At one level, these were infringements of the law, but neither neighbour wanted to pursue any legal proceedings. At another level, these episodes could be seen as the unacknowledged desire of the old lady to have some relationship with her neighbours and to escape from her self-imposed prison. Both her neighbours had family and friends and there was frequently laughter in their gardens. Perhaps the old lady wanted to possess and acquire something of their pleasure, but she wanted to acquire it without the years of work in making the relationships.

When my husband's personality was fragmenting there were occasions when he showed a breakdown in boundaries. Before he retired I used to travel to London frequently and paid for a personal car-parking space in a multi-storey car park in Inverness. After John had retired, and I used it less frequently, I was surprised one day to be told by the car-park attendant to move my car because that space belonged to Dr Forsythe. I said that I was Dr Forsythe but the attendant laughed and said 'You are hardly Dr John Forsythe'. (My husband was not a doctor.) On that occasion I assumed the confusion was a mistake. But in the years that followed I discovered that he had changed his name on many papers, including income tax forms. I think that this was part of an unconscious breaking down of his inner boundaries.

In the creation myth, the great world, or macrocosm, had the dry land distinguished from the undifferentiated waters. If one sees man as a small world, a microcosm, within the macrocosm, the dry land of his reasoning brain and conscious world needs to be distinguished from the deep water world of his depths or roots. However, if there is no communication between these two parts, pressure builds up and eventually the waters break through in an uncontrollable flood.

Water is a common symbol in people's dreams. Here is one. 'There is water coming through the front of my bedroom ceiling above the window, more than a trickle, and the ceiling is beginning to give way. I feel it is going to be a flood. I know where the stopcock in the kitchen is and that I can turn it off before damage is done. In the dream I know that it is a dream and that it will be all right.' There is no confusion here between the levels. The dreamer was able to look at the meaning of this dream and reorganise parts of her life, in a sense to turn off the stopcock, so that there was no flood of her conscious daytime mind by her night-time mind, part of her deep inner reality.

Another old lady, who was becoming confused, believed that she had water coming through her roof. She repeatedly telephoned a good-natured local builder to tell him about it. She asked him to go up on her roof and find where the water was coming in and stop it. He went to see her on many occasions, went up on the roof, did not find a leak and never charged her. She pointed at the floor and told him to look because the water was there, but he could not see it. One day she called him to say water was pouring from all the taps and they could not be turned off. He went, found all the taps had been turned full on and turned them off. She denied having turned them on, but this incident was repeated on a number of occasions. In one way, she was acting out a dream but it had no meaning for her and caused much work for somebody else. When the dreamer identified the levels, the meaning was, for her, productive and she could act to prevent any sort of flood; but for the confused old lady, whose inner boundaries were breaking down, there was no meaning in what she did.

Boundary wars

The person who dements is often highly intelligent, a capable manager and organiser. She may have lived life successfully in outer reality and laid great stress on being able to think everything out.

Each of the lives narrated here was lived with a considerable degree of competence at the outer, branch, level, but in each person there is evidence of a failure to be in touch with the deeper root level. The early lives and losses of each person in this book give an indication of the child's need to find a secure place in his private world over which he has control; that control was achieved to some degree through the powers of reason and intellectual achievement.

Each of these people has put great emphasis on the thinking and controlling part of themselves and has not taken any account of a possible other and opposite part. But suppose that each individual was not *either* the sort of person who paints, writes, and can very easily access the world of imagination *or* the sort of person who lives in the head and is governed by reason and logic. Suppose there is the potential for each individual to become a balanced person, and that in each of them there is the possibility of becoming *both* the thinking sort of person *and* the imaginative sort of person, although in any one individual one part may be predominant. There come rare moments in people's lives which offer the possibility of seeing and understanding something different and unusual for that particular person. I think that it is at these moments there is the possibility of taking on board this strange and unknown part, resurrecting it from the unperceived roots, becoming aware of messages from the depths. The root system within us is very dark, and it is an exquisitely difficult and painful process to listen to and accept messages from it; but the denial of these moments, the suppression of them, the slamming of the door on them, precipitates the retreat into disintegration. It is not deliberate and it is not conscious; but it is a blind refusal to accept. At the moment of retreat, other powerful forces take over and the responsibility for the individual's life is also handed over. If we refuse all these rather unexpected and strange gifts that can erupt from the roots we gradually lose contact with our depths and the source of our nourishment.

An individual who is at war within himself, whose boundaries are closed and who survives by suppressing the other side of himself, making reason his main value, appears to end up in a private hell. I look here at John, my husband, who had a very imaginative and creative father but who never wanted to know about this other part of himself. At the moment when his feeling and sensitive side showed itself, the door was slammed.

Reconciliation across the divide

Peace can never be imposed on inner war from outside; only when the opposites can be accepted is there hope. And there is a lot of accepting to be done. The losses that occur through the denial of the different parts of ourselves can be redeemed. The words 'redeemed' and 'redemption' have religious overtones, but the root meaning is 'to buy back'. There is no buying back on that level through material forces, or through the power of the intellect and its achievements; there is no redemption through reason. William Blake knew this very well when he wrote his lines on four-fold vision.

Now I a fourfold vision see,
And a fourfold vision is given to me;
'Tis fourfold in my supreme delight
And threefold in soft Beulah's night
And twofold Always. May God us keep
From single vision and Newton's sleep!
Buying back comes through the courage to open yourself

up to and accept unconditionally the total package which life offers you: the awe and the mystery, creative imagination, dreams, the things that come to us and overwhelm us and over which we have no control at all. It is a response from somewhere deep inside us that we do not program. And I spell 'program' here with one 'm' because I want to make it comparable to the world of computers. In that world we are in charge, we do the programming, we make the computer do what we want – if we can attain to sufficient know-how and are fortunate. (I speak with feeling because I am struggling to work with a new one and have considerable difficulty.) But my vision of integration in old age is the complete opposite of the world of computers. With a computer the aim is for me to be master, to have control; in the living of old age, of the bringing back, of the integration, a different part of me is at the centre. It is not the head bit of me that learns how to program the computer.

Through redemption can come a state of joy which is very different from being happy or content. That state can be induced in many ways, but joy is another of the gifts over which we have no control. Like the others, it comes with the option of acceptance or rejection. Making ourselves happy can be attempted with money, winning the lottery jackpot, bigger and better houses, more clothes, faster cars and the whole panoply of the material and secular Western world.

Blake sees single vision, the world of reason, as a terrible state in which to be; the best place is the world of the creative imagination. This is the world of fairy stories for children, or for adults, of reading novels or watching or listening to drama. This is the whole world of creative activity, of drawing, painting, writing poetry and making music. It might be described as a world of wasting time and doing nothing necessary, worthy or useful. I remember when I was a child that it was not accepted in our home that reading could be done before lunch. I used to try to become invisible in the back of a large armchair, so that I could disappear and go on reading. I was usually extricated from my retreat and sent to do something more useful. At this time I must have learned about an inner reality, or world of imagination. At that time I knew it was forbidden; now I know that it is of great value.

Helen Luke writes in her essays on old age, with reference to Eliot's poem *'Little Gidding'*:

The poet says he will disclose 'the gifts reserved for age' – the gifts that will crown his entire life. It is hard indeed as we reflect on the lines that these things are blessed gifts – gifts to be accepted in thankfulness if we are to fulfil the meaning of our lives.

The gifts are three. First, the changes taking place in the body – for some a sudden loss of physical health, or a gradual lessening of the energies which have flowed through the senses. Sight may grow dim, or hearing less acute; taste, smell and touch may lose their power to delight us. Many activities on which we have depended become impossible . . .

The second gift, says Eliot, is helpless rage at the terrifying folly of men and of their laughter at things which are not, we discover, even faintly amusing, but tragically serious. We cry out in frustrated horror at the blindness of those in political power; we see behind the exuberance of youth the shadow of violence or the excesses into which so many fall, and behind the beauty of romantic love the seeds of jealousy, possessiveness and hate; and we shrink at the laughter which is the joy of life, subtly decaying into the laughs that wound and pierce the dignity of man or woman. And so we may end through this rage identified with all that we rage against. This is a truth that becomes daily more evident as we watch the increasing intolerance of many who fight for good causes . . . Only the creative imagination in each of us finds the place beyond rage, which is truly compassion and the laughter of joy.

Third and last is the gift of memories, which in the old, grow stronger and more vivid as they look back over the story of their lives. If we are able to look at the past clear-eyed, we shall recognise how many of our acts and achievements which we thought virtuous, kind, and good, were also the cause of much harm to others.

CHAPTER 10

Shall I grow into old age or wither away?

It is a reasonable assumption that nobody wants to change or be changed. When money, control, power, establishment, position, property, success are involved, there will be strong resistance to any change at all. As with political parties, people may be willing to change the image, the message, the packaging, the innuendo, but in the end they will coerce and bribe to hang on to power and not change one item.

However, supposing we could stand aside for a few moments and watch this drama as a spectator who has nothing to lose by watching, we might see a different viewpoint. To suspend the habits of a lifetime for even one second is a difficult and intimidating challenge. There could be an immediate refusal. Having acknowledged the great difficulty of seeing a familiar thing in a different way, we can at least begin to understand all the influences of our past life that make us cling so tenaciously to the *status quo*. We have been conditioned since birth, been taught and have become accustomed, to seeing things in a certain conventional and established way. Now, while we are in a state of suspended belief, it will be interesting to consider a premise. Is it possible that health is different from the way in which it is currently understood at the end of the twentieth century? Just supposing there is a power, a creator, a designer, who is far greater than man's comprehension and unable to be encompassed by man's intellect, and this power thinks with other thoughts and abilities, and speaks in another language.

Further, suppose that within each human being there is a minuscule portion of this greater power which can only make contact with, or become in any way in relationship with, this overall great power when man's assumed control is limited and his resistance to losing his own control is diminished. But the stronger a man's intellect, organisation, power and control over himself and the universe in which he spends his life, the more difficult it is for the contact between the over-riding great power and the minuscule inner bit in every man to get in touch with each other.

Suppose that health meant a state of wholeness, or even holiness, and suppose this wholeness is a balance between control and loss of control, inner and outer realities, and that the overall design is that each human should complete this final balance before death. The loss of control requisite for such a balance can either happen through man's choice and free will, with surrender of his control, in which case it happens with meaning, or it happens without man's choice, in spite of himself, in which case it happens without meaning.

There is a current delusion that the great overall power is nice and kind, a benevolent father figure who wants only our happiness. But could this be a fallacy? If we dare to assume that the great overall power desires that each minuscule microcosm should, in some way beyond man's understanding, become a mirror image of the great macrocosm of all that is created, could it follow that the microcosm also has to take on, in diminished form, all the opposites of light and dark, night and day, heaven and earth, loving and hating, sickness and health, chaos and order, destruction and creation? For the superorganised person who has everything under control, the opposite is chaos, disorder, confusion, complete loss of control, weakness and all the things which he has tried, during his whole life, to wall up and keep at a distance; a veritable Pandora's box of horrors with every sort of disgusting filth in all its nooks and crannies. For the organiser, the problem solver, this scenario is disaster; he will attempt to fill any empty space with another set of things over which he does have control. But could all the confusion and muck be the raw materials, the building blocks, for those who are prepared to be in touch with the part of themselves that is creative and artistic? They could see this load of old discarded rubbish as a gift. Here there is an echo from the alchemists who attempted to produce gold from base metals.

The opposite of organisation and control is confusion and weakness. If you choose to surrender control, which is very difficult, there will be a sense of loss and confusion; but in the end there can be a new comprehension of meaning far beyond any possible expectation, and ultimately a greater hope of wholeness. If surrender is refused, ultimately it is imposed, which leads to confusion and no understanding or meaning.

Suppose we do get what we most desire in life, but it is given to us with so much camouflage that it is unrecognisable. On the theme of the things we want, and the manner in which we see them as curse or blessing, this prayer is a summary:

So easily do we pray for the wrong things:

For strength that we may achieve, and God gives us weakness that we may be humble;

For health that we may do great things, and God gives us infirmity that we may do better things;

For riches that we may be happy, and God gives us
poverty that we may be wise;
For power that we may have the praise of men, and God
gives us weakness that we may feel the need of him;
For all things that we may have life, and God gives us life
that we may enjoy all things.
And so having received nothing that we have asked for
but all things that we have genuinely hoped for, our
prayer has been answered, and we have been blessed.

The person who has always most desired control over
himself, those around him and his immediate vicinity may
indeed get it. That could be a picture of Alzheimer's disease,
where the patient does have control, but forgoes all responsibility and is robbed of any sense of meaning in his life.
Being made whole, in the widest sense, is prevented by the
need for control; some people are unwilling to relinquish
one tiny bit of that power to control. There is a price to pay
for health or wholeness and most people do not want, or do
not see the need, to pay it. At a physical level, the price may
be as straightforward as giving up smoking to avoid lung
cancer, giving up alcohol, losing weight, sticking to a diet,
leading a more orderly life, but against this there is the
demand for comfort; and the demand becomes a need and
satisfaction may be supplied.

Sometimes, losing control can mean giving up the use of
an illness to control other people. Sickness is a powerful
weapon and can be used to massive effect. If the gains are
great enough, the use of illness is encouraged and its per-
petuation guaranteed. The more that is invested in the illness, and the greater the need of the patient for the illness,
the stronger will be the hold of the illness over the patient.
When weakness is acknowledged and accepted, many

changes can take place, but when the same weakness is turned around and used as a weapon, there is increased control and less possibility of that person becoming whole.

All those whose stories are in this book are good, hardworking and essentially conformist people. They were all, for one reason or another, forced into a position early in life of taking over control of their lives. Each one had to use all the power at his disposal in order to survive. In 1887 Lord Acton wrote 'Power tends to corrupt, and absolute power corrupts absolutely'. In the *Dictionary of Word Origins* the word 'corrupt' is derived from the Latin verb *rumpere* meaning 'to break'. 'It entered into partnership with the intensive prefix com— to produce corrumpere "destroy completely."' And the word 'absolute', from the same dictionary, in this sense, means 'free from any qualification or restriction'. The exercise of power occurs within the person, and the domination is that of the reason over the roots of feeling and instinct.

The moment when somebody is stripped of the facade, a woman loses her husband or health, a man loses his job or retires, are seen as totally unacceptable losses because of the values of this world. Then the loss can become an illness, be given a name, put into the hands of the doctors. Responsibility is handed over, the illness is investigated, and can then assume power and prestige. Each of the losses or failures has the potential to be the balancing factor, a means of becoming more whole; but each one, when it takes over and has power invested in it, becomes a further means of destruction and fragmentation. Each loss or failure leaves an empty space which is seen either as the potential for something creative to occur, or as a threat which is rapidly filled up. It is difficult to leave the spaces because they seem like little deaths, forerunners of final death, the loss of everything at the outer level. But an ongoing death is not a disaster. It is a strange and new experience and there are moments of joy. We have no control over death and we cannot confine death to the chronological moment of dying. Death is much wider than that moment. It may be the refusal to die daily, to let go and give up all our possessions of various kinds, that expedites a disintegration.

For the majority of people the time comes, either rapidly or gradually, when many losses, weaknesses and failures are experienced. All the roles that have made them important crumble and disappear. We can be left suspended between a dependent childhood, a long phase of role-playing, and the prospect of old age and death. We may not realise what is happening. At one level, it is easier to carry on in the way in which we have always lived our lives, denying that there is any change, filling any chink in the space with activity. The alternative is to stop, recognise and understand the profound changes that are occurring, and become aware of alternative ways of living. Disintegration could be precipitated at the moment when we lose our many roles, but fail to see the meaning and importance of the loss.

Helen Luke writes in her essay on *The Tempest*,

At the end of the play Prospero had said that henceforth every third thought of his would be of his grave. But that, in old age, may be a sign of the very opposite of despair, arising from the growing recognition of death as woven into the fabric of any life that has meaning; indeed such frequent attention to the meaning of death may be the way to the final release from the shadow of despair. Having made that remark about death he bids Ariel see to giving the ships 'calm seas, auspicious gales'. Then he stands, stripped of all his powers, suddenly face to face with the realisation of what lies before him, and of what it really means to forgive and be forgiven and so to be ready to die.

It is a strange paradox that the acceptance of losses can lead to a great coming together within a person; but the hanging on, refusal to let go, of all the roles, possessions and outer trappings of life, can lead to disintegration. An acceptance of the loss of home, spouse, money, or professional role can also lead to release from the fear of death. This can bring a sense of freedom and hope. The few things that are left at that point are ones that nobody can remove by the exercise of any worldly power.

Busy-ness is one way of compensating for losses. It can look good to onlookers and make the person feel important and valuable. The alternative to living in a straight line is to stop, look hard, begin to see the profound changes that are happening, and dare to discover other ways of living the remainder of our lives. Disintegration could begin, in an already prone personality, at the moment when we lose our many roles, but fail to understand the significance of the loss. If we have lived secure in the belief that what we do is who we are, it is appallingly difficult to drop off the all important 'doing' bit of us.

After the death of somebody from Alzheimer's disease, the bereaved carer is in a similar position. She may have lost an important role as carer at the moment when she is already battered by the experience of living close to somebody else's disintegration. At these moments of loss there is the opportunity to look beyond the playing of roles, a time to explore and develop our own hidden potential.

The second half or third or quarter of life, if we have set our values in the 'having' mode, is a serial loss and deprivation, with no possibility of any compensatory gain.

My health may go, and also my job and my money. My husband may die, my children have left home, my fertility will go or have been taken away by a hysterectomy, and so on. As old age approaches, many people do become poorer, give up professional status and power, move to smaller homes and even have to give up their car! We give up all these possessions either with good grace, possibly even with thankfulness, or we hang on to them with ever decreasing credibility, or we have them snatched from us while we protest loudly. The loss of all or any of our possessions can cause great sadness; the amount of sadness will be proportional to the degree of our belief that these were necessary and integral parts of our value. If the size of our house and the road in which it is sited are vital parts of our personal value, their loss or diminution also devalues us as persons.

Bereavement can be an opportunity for accepting a 'mid-life' crisis. Most of us have spent the first fifty years or so of our life entrenched in the 'having' mode, backed up by a culture that favours and supports this mode. It is, therefore, extremely difficult to accept all these losses as anything but failure. Only in a change of the person from the 'having' mode to the 'being' mode can such losses be understood as anything but bereavement, robbery of what we have seen as ours by right. But the loss of the need for the possessions, not necessarily the loss of the actual possessions, can lead to a kind of liberation and ultimately to joy.

The myth of Orpheus and Eurydice, from a time long past but always present and relevant, illustrates what I try to say. Eurydice, Orpheus's wife and great love, was killed by the bite of a serpent and was taken into the underworld. Orpheus, through the power of his lyre-playing, manages to find her and eventually receives permission to take her back to earth, on one condition. He must not look back at her. He starts out on their journey back, and Eurydice follows him, but there comes a moment when he is unable to trust that his lover is still there. He looks back to make sure, to know that he can repossess her, and at that moment she is taken back into the underworld and lost to him for ever.

Psychosomatic disease

Psychosomatic disease is a description applied to many modern diseases and is often used without a full understanding of what the words mean. By definition a psychosomatic disease is one of the *psyche* and the *soma*. *Psyche*, from the Greek, means 'breath, soul, spirit' as distinct from the body. During the nineteenth century, the word meaning changed a little to mean 'mind' and thus 'psychiatry' came to mean a way of healing conditions of the mind. *Soma* means 'the body'. Although 'psychosomatic' means 'of the body and the spirit or mind', it is all too often misconstrued into meaning '*either* body *or* mind'. 'This illness of mine is definitely physical and not all in my mind' is often said; there are physical changes so this disease cannot be psychosomatic. But if the dis-ease is of both psyche and soma, it is surely inevitable that there will be changes in both the psyche and the soma. A change in understanding from either/or to also/and is always a difficult leap into the unknown.

During the past fifty years there have been a number of outbreaks of mysterious disease, for example the so-called Royal Free Disease in the 1950s, whose origins have been disputed. Some have said there is a physical cause, but there have been difficulties in demonstrating it. Others have said they are outbreaks of mass hysteria. The word 'hysteria' comes from the Greek word *husterikos* meaning 'suffering in the womb'. During the nineteenth century the word hysteria was used to describe a condition occurring in women which was also known as 'the vapours' and was considered a neurosis.

If we attempt a mental leap into the unknown, and look at hysteria not as a 'neurotic' condition applying to a woman's mind, but in a more general sense as suffering in the womb, and then relate this to the mythology of the earth mother in the dark underworld, the great root system of mankind, could these diseases be construed as springing from the darkness of each individual and then spreading within society through the interconnected root systems? Then we could postulate that such conditions could develop without the knowledge or understanding of the branches of mankind. There could be an intolerable stress between the dark and hidden world of the roots and the world of the tree that is visible in the light of day and of reason.

The word stress is part of everyday parlance and it can mean anything from anxiety about paying the next tele-phone bill to an argument with a partner, from a bereave-ment to a divorce. It is assumed by doctor and patient alike that there will be a recognisable and articulated reason for the stress before a medical condition associated with stress can be diagnosed. However, if the invisible root system is accepted as an integral part of the person, there could be stresses between the conscious mind, which can be recog-nised, and the unconscious mind, which could be out of bounds for the conscious mind. There could also be stresses within the unconscious mind between drives that want one sort of outcome and forces which want the opposite. None of these forces are accessible to the conscious mind. This conflict, which is totally at an unconscious level, might only become apparent by some signal which is easily recognisable by the conscious mind. It can then be labelled and appropriate action taken. An alarm signal is sent from the roots to make the tree above ground aware of something important for its survival. Perhaps the disintegration that occurs in dementia occurs at a moment when it is most difficult for the outer self, with its roles and goals and possessions and demands for control and organisation, and the unknown, frail and secret inner self, to hold together as one single integrated entity. If the outer reality has always been all-important, any changes in it may be overpowering for somebody with a poor sense of their own inner reality.

The awe and the mystery

During my travels, meeting relatives and carers of those who have developed Alzheimer's disease, I have heard the words 'awe and mystery' used on many occasions. They have not been used in an overtly religious context or by people who have any connection with the organised church; but awe and mystery have been identified as valuable concepts that have disappeared from the contemporary world.

On one occasion the words occurred during a talk with friends in California. One woman in the group had a mother developing Alzheimer's disease, and another had a mother who had died from it. We were all connected with creative activities, writers, a musician, a dancer. During the conversation the words awe and mystery were spoken of as missing in the emotional climate of contemporary California.

Later in the day we were in a redwood forest. It was

September and there were few holiday-makers around. We left the car and walked along duckboards into a remote part of the forest to look at one particular large tree. We stood a few feet away from each other, in silence. For minutes there was no sound. The great trees around us, with their riven trunks and peeling bark, in all their sombre colours of brown and blue and green, were awe-inspiring. They were about fourteen hundred years old. I thought of the wooden Saxon churches in England built at the time the trees were saplings. They had the same sense of holiness.

Suddenly the silence was broken by the sound of crackling leaves about twenty yards away up a small incline. We all shifted our positions a little to look. The sound was repeated and then, in the light from a shaft from the sun through the foliage, we saw a deer and then another and another moving through the forest.

Here were the awe and the mystery. In busy lives, time and energy had been found to go there and be still and silent.

Creative imagination

Everybody can write and paint. Not everybody is a genius but the potential is always there. However, there is also the bit in every man that says 'No, I can't write or paint and as for being a poet, think again'. I do not believe that this person has no creative imagination or artistic talent. I think that, at an early age, they have been crushed and a bit of the person who did the crushing has been implanted in the victim, and thrived and grown so strong that as soon as a drawing is started, the crusher raises a disparaging voice and says, 'That's no good, at all. You ought to spend your time doing something useful.' There is another killing voice of patronage that goes something like this, 'That's a clever picture dear,' or, 'What a nice poem, isn't she clever?' Those remarks mean death to the emergence and growth of the smallest spark of creative spirit.

In older age it does not matter if we achieve anything or not. We can challenge the destructive voices if we desire to sufficiently. Everybody can write; it is irrelevant whether the material is published or not. Everybody can draw and paint; again it is irrelevant if the paintings are exhibited and sold or not. Fun is the aim, if there must be a stated intention. It is not a question of learning how to do things, going to classes, or taking courses to learn how to write poetry or paint properly for the approval of the crusher; but of daring to be still with oneself and play with pencils, paints and paper, and write what comes and paint what arrives. It is the playing, without any desire for achievement, that is vital at this stage of life. How sad that, at the present time in the UK, adult education is increasingly geared to achievement and awards are made for attendance at courses.

If we go from one sort of achieving to another, we have not changed direction and are still living in outer reality. It is the people who know, in Denis Healey's word, their 'hinterland', who can walk in the dark woods of their inmost being, in solitude, and eventually not be frightened of the darkness and find individual treasures in the depths of the roots, who will not disintegrate.

The world of the imagination can feel like a threat to those who have lived in the world of outer reality and relied on their own power of reason to keep control. Any glimpse of this underworld of the imagination may be a great threat because, if imagination is allowed to develop, it is the beginning of loss of conscious control. I believe that fear of the imagination can trigger a response to keep the hatch closed, to slam the door to the underworld, because we are never in control of our imagination. Those who have lived close to somebody who has disintegrated may be able to identify the moment at which the door to the underworld has slammed.

I remember the empty space, and see more clearly that allowing the emptiness to be guarded for the work of creative imagination does not mean living in a state of chaos and disorder. Much hard work and discipline is necessary to keep the boundaries to your space, or it will be taken over by a multiplicity of worthy activities. We must find a secure time and a private place to give the creative sparks the opportunity to grow. The potting shed at the end of the garden is a good sanctuary; a proper place for creative pottering. Pottering has both active and passive origins. The pot is the cup, the holder of the elixir, the acceptance of the whole; and another reminder of the work of the alchemists with their retort in which they heated base metals. Pottering also means the making of the pots; pottering is both the doing and the receiving. The potting shed, where cuttings can be taken and put in good soil and watered regularly while one waits for new growth, is a good place for such creative activity.

In earlier times a woman had her boudoir for withdrawal during certain hours each day. Older age can provide the opportunity to reclaim such a privilege. The place does not need to be a literal potting shed or boudoir; but it needs to have a well-defined boundary and to be quiet and secluded. When I am on my own in my kitchen, preparing simple food, I can find the essence of the boudoir. To be on one's own at a regular interval, in a certain place and at a certain time, helps to develop an inner peace and better relationship with one's own roots. In the last years of life it is important, because being born into this world and the departure from this world through death are both solitary journeys, whatever helping hands are present.

Social activities, watching television and organised games make no demand on nor do they nourish the inner world of creative imagination. They can be good recreations in limited amounts but as a major part of the daily mental and emotional diet they can lead to a nutritionally deprived inner world and starvation of the roots.

Helen Luke, in her essay on *King Lear*, writes,

'So we'll live,' he continues. The exchange of blessings between one human being and another is the essence of life itself. 'And pray, and sing, and tell old tales, and laugh at gilded butterflies.' Here are the proper occupations of old age: prayer, which is the quickening of the mind, the rooting of the attention in the ground of being; song, which is the expression of joy in the harmony of the chaos; 'the telling of old tales', which among all primitives was the supreme function of the old, who passed on the wisdom of the ancestor through the symbol, through the understanding of the dreams of the race that their long experience had taught them. In our days how sadly lost, despised even, is the function of the old! Wisdom being identified with knowledge, the 'old tale' has become the subject of learned historical research, and only for the few does it remain the carrier of true wisdom of heart and mind, of body and spirit. When the old cease to 'dream dreams', to be 'tellers of tales', the time must come of which the Book of Proverbs speaks: 'Where there is no vision, the people perish.'

And laughter! Surely laughter of a certain kind springs from the heart of those who have truly grown old. It is the laughter of pure delight in beauty – beauty of which the golden butterfly is the perfect symbol – a fleeting, ephemeral thing, passing on the wind, eternally reborn from the earthbound worm, the fragile yet omnipotent beauty of the present moment.

All these four things are activities without purpose; any one of them is immediately killed by any hint of striving for achievement.

The dream is the most reliable messenger between roots and branches. I believe it is important to be more aware of our dreams in later life because they give us the symbols which hold the roots and branches of our lives together. If they are written down regularly it becomes easier to remember them. Painting, drawing or writing a poem about them will help us to understand this new language. Dreams are very private and should not be talked about, but it can help if there is one person with whom you can speak about them.

If we take this world of the dream seriously, it is important that we live in the best way possible to be aware of our dreams. Some drugs, such as sleeping pills and antidepressants, can impair the waking awareness of dreams. The drugs may be necessary as 'first aid' but should, when possible, be avoided on a long term basis. They can inhibit some symptoms which are distressing but may, at the same time and by the same means, inhibit a deeper awareness of the whole person. Each individual, if he puts his mind to it, can discover the best conditions to remember his dreams. A lot of noise and talking during the evening, too much television, alcohol in excess, extreme fatigue, are all things which may affect some people.

Loss of possessions

In the Funeral Service from *The Book of Common Prayer*, the following words are said as the priest walks in front of the coffin up the aisle of the church, 'We brought nothing into this world, and it is certain we can carry nothing out'. Nobody disputes the ultimate reality that we all shall die but how difficult it is at any age to let go daily.

When I feel threatened or under any pressure, I want to hang on to every little bit of what I see as mine, and attempt to keep it under my control. When I look again at the deep meaning of bereavement, robbery, and see every incident in my life as some sort of possession which can be taken away, I am more aware of the burden of possessiveness and the futility of my attempts to regain control over what has gone. If I am able to open my hands and let it go as thistledown upon the wind I regain all my sense of adventure and fun. I can only be robbed of what I possess or think that I possess. We cannot go back and relive any part of our life; and there come moments when it is necessary to shed another piece into a private wastepaper basket.

If we cannot accept the whole package that life gives us, we can fall into the habit of an 'if only' acceptance and we may put strange and unexpected conditions on life. 'If only I could just go on gardening I would go on living' or, 'If only I could be sure that this pain would not come back I might want to go on living.' These are phrases we have all heard, and how reasonable they are, but they are all imposing some sort of condition on life. There is a failure to accept present reality, and instead a fantasy of what could or might be a better reality. Conditional living could immunise us to seeing the joys of the present reality, joys as simple as the pattern of frost on the window glass or a spider's web sprinkled with snow.

The controlling mind, which has demanded that everything lost must be replaced, is confused by an irreplaceable loss. Charles Morgan wrote, in his novel *The Fountain*, 'When loss becomes freedom we are baptised in wonder and are fit to die.' In Helen Luke's writing on the novels of Charles Williams she quotes 'a very beautiful prayer in the *American New Episcopal Liturgy* which is said immediately after the symbolic immersion of baptism. In it are these words, "Sustain (him or her) O Lord, in your Holy Spirit. Give him an inquiring and discerning heart, the courage to will and to persevere, a spirit to know and to love you, and the gift of joy and wonder in all your works."' The prayer is written for the baptism of infants, but it seems to me to set out all the required qualities to dare to go on living into old age, with the dispossession of every inessential trapping and encumbrance.

The interval

Interval means the space between two walls; that too could be a boundary. I started this quest for the meaning of Alzheimer's disease ten years ago from a background of medical training and the experience of John's sickness. I accept all the scientific knowledge and medical understanding about this tragic condition, but in my searching I have had glimmers of other meanings of a different sort. I have not found answers to my questions but have discovered new ways of questioning. Unlike a mystery thriller writer, I am not able to produce the perpetrator of the crime. Now I shall rest in my personal search until I start the next endeavour.

Useful addresses

Age Concern England, Astral House, 1268 London Road, London SW16 4EJ. Tel. 0181 679 8000
Age Concern Scotland, 54a Fountain Bridge, Edinburgh EH3 9PT. Tel. 0131 228 5656
Age Concern Wales, 4th Floor, 1 Cathedral Street, Cardiff CF1 9SD. Tel. 01222 371 566
Age Concern Northern Ireland, 3 Lower Crescent, Belfast BT7 1NR. Tel. 01232 245 729

England
Alzheimer's Disease Society, Gordon House, 10 Greencoat Place, London SW1P 1PH. Tel. 0171 306 0606

Scotland
Alzheimer's Disease Society, 8 Hill Street, Edinburgh EH2 3JZ. Tel. 0131 225 1453

Wales
Alzheimer's Disease Society, Tonna Hospital, Neath, West Glamorgan SA11 3LX. Tel. 01639 641 939

Northern Ireland
Alzheimer's Disease Society, 11 Wellington Park, Belfast BT9 6DJ. Tel. 01232 664 100

Australia
Alzheimer's Disease and Related Disorders, PO Box 51, North Ryde, NSW 2113. Tel. 611 878 4466

USA
Alzheimer's Disease International, 70 East Lake Street, Chicago,
Illinois 60601-5997. Tel. 312 853 3060

Canada
Alzheimer's Society of Canada, 1320 Yonge Street, Suite 302,
Toronto, Ontario MJ4T 1X2. Tel. 416 925 3552

Association of Community Health Councils for England and
Wales, 30 Drayton Park, London N5 1PB. Tel. 0171 609 8405

Association of Crossroads Care Attendant Schemes, 10 Regent
Place, Rugby, Warwickshire CV21 2PN. Tel. 01788 573 653

British Red Cross Society, 9 Grosvenor Crescent, London
SW1X 7EJ. Tel. 0171 235 5454

Carers' National Association, 20/25 Glasshouse Yard, London
EC1A 4JS. Tel. 0171 490 8818

Court of Protection, 25 Store Street, London WC1E 7BP.
Tel. 0171 636 6877

Scotland
Court of Session, Meldrum House, 15 Drumsheugh Gardens,
Edinburgh EH3 3QG

Mind (National Association for Mental Health),
Granta House, 15-19 Broadway, Stratford, London E15 4BQ.
Tel. 0181 519 2122

National Association of Citizens Advice Bureaux, 115-123
Pentonville Road, London N1 9LZ. Tel. 0171 833 2181

Index